THE FLYING DOCTOR

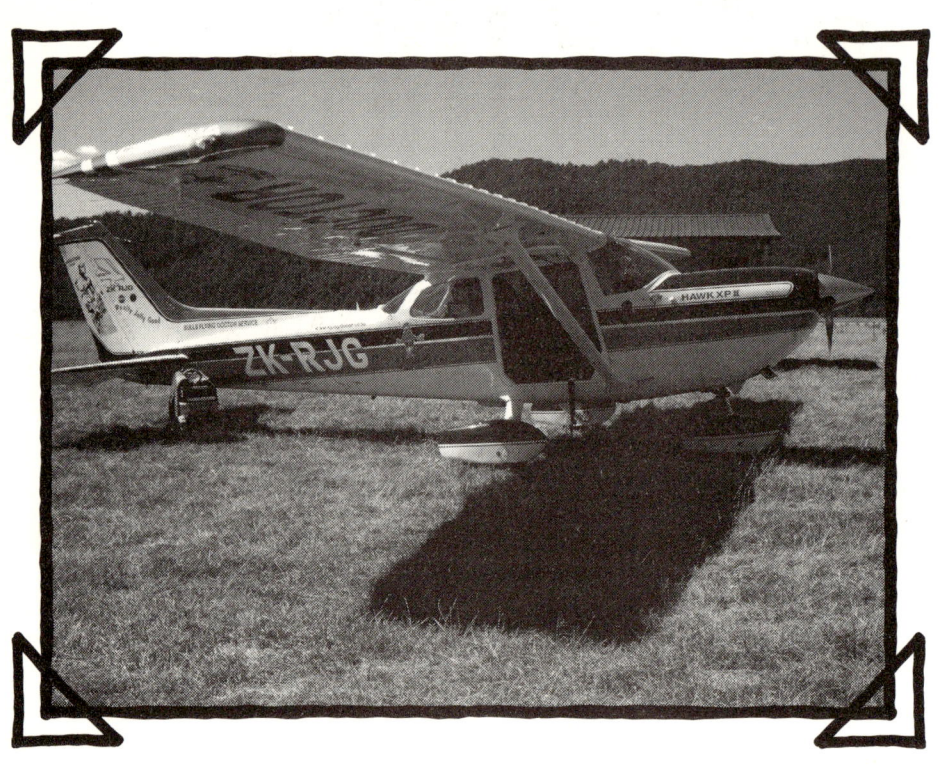

THE FLYING DOCTOR

DAVE BALDWIN

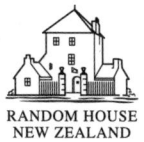

RANDOM HOUSE
NEW ZEALAND

To Marc

And so you've left us,
Journeyed off and soared aloft
To heights we can but dream.
God lent you for a little while,
Blessed us with your sunshine smile
And earthquake of a handshake,
Rattling every hangar's beam.
You need no rotors turning now
To lift you high in the cloudless sky —
Chopper pilot flying free
On eagles' wings eternally.
Our love goes with you and our pain,
Who knows when we'll meet you again?
Wherever turbines burn the air
We know your spirit's hovering there,
We sense you close in heart and prayer,
At peace.

— Raewyn Holden

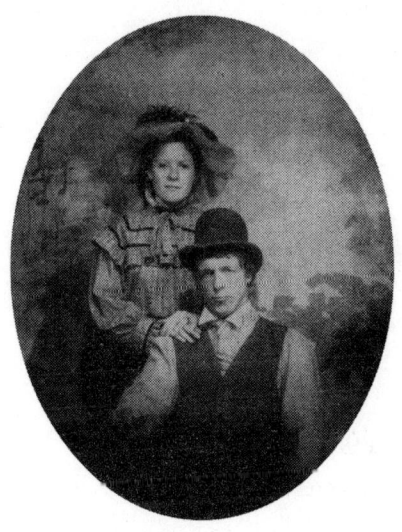

This book is dedicated to the best wife, mother and grandmother ever — Sandi Baldwin

RANDOM HOUSE

UK | USA | Canada | Ireland | Australia
India | New Zealand | South Africa | China

Random House is an imprint of the Penguin Random House group of companies, whose addresses can be found at global.penguinrandomhouse.com.

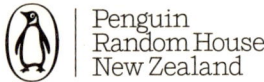

First published by Penguin Random House New Zealand, 2016

10 9 8 7 6 5 4 3 2 1

Text and photography © Dave Baldwin, 2016

The moral right of the author has been asserted.

All rights reserved. Without limiting the rights under copyright reserved above, no part of this publication may be reproduced, stored in or introduced into a retrieval system, or transmitted, in any form or by any means (electronic, mechanical, photocopying, recording or otherwise), without the prior written permission of both the copyright owner and the above publisher of this book.

Cover and text design by Sam Bunny © Penguin Random House New Zealand
Cover photograph by Mike Heydon/Jet Productions
Printed and bound in Australia by Griffin Press, an Accredited ISO AS/NZS 14001 Environmental Management Systems Printer

A catalogue record for this book is available from the National Library of New Zealand.

ISBN 978-1-77553-892-9
eISBN 978-1-77553-893-6

penguin.co.nz

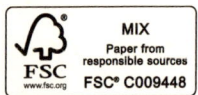

CONTENTS

Introduction		9
Chapter 1	Yearning for freedom	17
Chapter 2	Time to get me some schooling	33
Chapter 3	I culd not spel dokta but now I are one	55
Chapter 4	Horsepital here we come	77
Chapter 5	The soldier in me	95
Chapter 6	My destiny is in Bulls	117
Chapter 7	Freedom is coming	137
Chapter 8	The Bulls Flying Doctor Service is born	153
Chapter 9	Becoming respectable	173
Chapter 10	Maturing as an organisation	193
Chapter 11	A few West Coast tales	213
Chapter 12	Trials and tribulations	235
Chapter 13	Au revoir, Marc	253
Chapter 14	Beyond the material world	269
Epilogue		281
Acknowledgements		285

INTRODUCTION

It was Sax — Dave Saxton — who originally introduced me to the term 'Godzone'. I knew exactly what he meant, and I am reminded of it, over and over again, on trips like this one.

I've just left Christchurch-controlled airspace — I signed off by assuring the controller that I would have my first whitebait patty in her honour — and I'm now cruising at 10,000 feet on visual flight rules (VFR) over the headwaters of the Rakaia River. The weather is sparkling clear, with only a few shreds of cloud around good old Cloud Piercer, Aoraki/Mount Cook, which is, of course, busy piercing them. The other big fellas — Malte Brun, Tasman, Dampier — stand close by, too. The terrain repeatedly soars to meet me and then plunges away — scree slopes, fields of golden tussock, icefalls, jewel-like tarns.

You may have heard of Dave Saxton. He's one of the legends of the aviation scene around South Westland and Fiordland, a part of the world where there is no shortage of legends, characters, colourful individuals and downright dangerous bastards. There's a story about him — there's actually a few stories about Sax — where he was returning from a trip north with a couple of mates. He paused at the head of the gangway of the Interislander, swept an arm to take in the South Island, and said to his mates: 'There you go, boys. The winter block.' As with 'Godzone', I know exactly what he meant and I know exactly what he was feeling when he said it. The South Island is God's Own Country, all right; a playground for anyone who loves the outdoors. It's always good to be back.

ZK-Really-Jolly-Good, my Cessna 172 Hawk XP2, bounces around in the thermals at the head of the Godley River valley, and I brace by gripping the bit of Arawata River schist velcroed to the top of the instrument panel as a handpiece. Lake Tekapo is spread out ahead of me, the kind of pastel blue that was fashionable in the 1930s. Shortly it'll be time to let the local pilots who are flying in the vicinity of Wanaka know that I'm inbound. My eye roves over the instruments out of habit: fuel good in both tanks, leaning just right. All good.

I'm a bit shagged, truth be told. I was on call all morning at my medical practice across the way at Bulls in the lower North Island, and got away much later in the afternoon than I usually aim to. So while I'm keeping an eye on the plane, I'm also keeping an eye on myself. Just to be sure, I reach across to the thermos I have in a holder on the starboard side of the cockpit and pour myself a cup of weapons-grade coffee, white and sweetened with just a dash of my favourite borage honey from the Nimmos' farm in the Clarence River valley.

South of the Mackenzie Country, parts of the mighty

INTRODUCTION

Landsborough River valley are in view. I can't look at this area without a grin and a pang. It's where me, my best mate and son Marc, and my mum, Granny Olive, used to come to hunt the roar as the 'Gang of Three'.

Great times.

Every one of my trips south is a sentimental journey. As my GPS ticks off waypoints along the route I've logged into it, my soul kind of does the same thing. I have a photo of the Gang of Three on our first roar trip, where Marc bagged his first stag at the age of nine: it seems stupid that I'm the only one of us still right side up. I dip a wing to my ghosts and carry on.

Quite recently, I made the decision that The Not-So-Royal Bulls Flying Doctor Service wasn't going to do rotary-wing aircraft (or, as they're rather better known, 'choppers'). Plenty of people have told me I'm mad doing what I do with a fixed-wing, but after 16 years and 3500 hours of flying I know this little plane backwards. Instead of going for a rotary-wing rating and getting hold of a chopper, I decided I would invest in some big wheels and vortex generators for Really-Jolly-Good. The wheels slow me down — the GPS indicates I'm probably losing a good 10 knots in speed over the ground at 10,000 feet — but as I say to people, it means I simply spend longer in paradise. And man, do those big tyres smooth out the bumps on some of the more tricky strips I land on. The vortex generators — a series of little fins mounted behind the leading edges of the wings, the tailfin and tailplane — have really improved the short take-off and landing capabilities of my little aircraft, turning it into a poor man's helicopter. I'm happy with that.

Plus, I can't even handle T-Rex, the floor polisher at our

medical practice, so what hope would I have of landing a chopper in a tight bush clearing? You've got to be pretty sharp. I've lost so many good mates in chopper crashes lately, good bastards who knew what they were doing.

I give the local pilots a heads-up on 119.1 MHz and 120.1 MHz that I'm descending to land at Wanaka Airport, doing a big arc over the Clutha in its plush golden terraces. It's beautiful country: I never get tired of this place. There's another plane about; I can't see him, but he's happy to go number two, to join the circuit and land behind me. There's a paraglider somewhere — Aha! Got you, you bastard, over there, by the outlet on the edge of Lake Hawea. So I'm all set to land. I line up. It's been a hot day, and the plane wobbles a bit on approach, but I get her on the tarmac nice and sweet with a little bump and squeak of my new tyres.

I taxi in and park next to the fuel bowsers. I've got a few medicals to do here, in the Wanaka Aerospace Research Institute in the Wallis boys' Alpine Helicopters buildings. The first of the pilots is there already, leaning on the fence and wearing a big grin. I reckon he's impressed by my big new wheels.

When I take off again for the 40-minute flight to Te Anau, it's as though a weight has been lifted from my shoulders. After the morning's on-call load and four medical inspections back there in Wanaka, I'm buggered and ready for a beer. The chances of not getting one at Noddy Deaker's place — the Upukerora Aerospace Research Institute — are absolutely zero, I'd say.

INTRODUCTION

The sun is low as I transit Queenstown's tightly controlled airspace. You have to do everything by the book with these buggers, because it's a tricky place to fly in anything, let alone the big planes they get in and out of here, so they're sticklers. I wind the controller up a bit about the prospect of night flights starting up soon. I hope he gets to be a rich man from all the pending overtime, I tell him, and offer to help him out if he ever ends up having too much money.

Approaching the Von River valley, I remind myself to keep my wits about me. Looking into the setting sun can make you miss subtleties in the terrain, and just because I've flown this route dozens of times doesn't mean I can afford to be complacent. The mountain shadows can easily hide an oncoming ridge, and bang! It's all over, rover! Finally out of the mountains, I fly through Bald Pass, always a highlight on this leg. That panoramic view of Lake Te Anau and Fiordland National Park suddenly comes into view and it's to die for.

The weather has remained flawless, with just a thin veil of mist creeping towards the southern reaches of Lake Te Anau from Manapouri. I have perfect conditions to land at Noddy's. I do a pass and waggle my wings, and then slip down to make my final. It's a shortish strip, approached by sinking through a shelter belt of poplars and a low hedge. It's slightly downhill over the smooth grass; get it wrong and you'll not only collect a deer fence but most likely end up in the living room of Noddy and Sue's lovely new home.

But I get it right, and Dick (Noddy's older brother) is already opening the big gates for me so I can taxi to a halt in front of the hangar that houses the Upukerora Aerospace Research Institute.

Dick's another legend from these parts. He's one of the most experienced helicopter pilots in the country, and most of that experience was gained in the venison recovery business. He and Noddy have been a team for the best part of 50 years, and Noddy has shot over 100,000 deer, mostly from Dick's machine. Good bastards, the pair of them. I'm lucky to get to spend my time in this sort of company.

'How you doing, you bastard?' Dick greets me, as I wind the prop down.

'Not telling, but I could murder a beer,' I say.

'No chance,' he laughs. 'Just finished the last ice-cold stubby, and jeez it was good!'

Dinner is roast lamb and veges that Noddy and Sue have grown themselves, including some sweet white turnips that Noddy's daughter sent up from down by Invercargill. There is a cold beer, after all, and in the morning there's wild mushrooms on toast. I've got 10 medicals to do, which takes me till midday.

Noddy has gone off to play with a digger down at Manapouri, but when I'm finally ready to leave Dick's there to see me off. The day began with a thick fog blanketing everything, so you couldn't even see through to the Jackson Peaks across the way. Noddy promised it would be gone by now, and he's obviously had a word with the authorities. Another sparklingly fine day, my work over and nothing in prospect but an afternoon spent in the company of the mountains, the tahr and chamois and my memories.

INTRODUCTION

I open the throttle on Really-Jolly-Good, manage not to collect the deer fence or end up watching daytime TV in the Deakers' living room and soar into the air with the roar of full power.

Christ, I think. I'm doing it. I'm living the dream. I couldn't want for anything, could I? Or only one thing.

CHAPTER 1

YEARNING FOR FREEDOM

I was born and grew up in the North Island, but my folks were Mainlanders. Olive Garraway was 26 when she met Alfred Charles Gordon 'Stan' Baldwin, who was 55. Besides cradle-snatching, Stan was an expert in aircraft instruments and had immigrated to New Zealand just before the outbreak of the Second World War to take up a position as an instructor in instrument repair, calibration and maintenance for the Royal New Zealand Air Force (RNZAF).

Stan met Olive in 1953 at the Taieri Air Force Base where he was stationed. The airbase was attached to the RNZAF flight school, where Olive was assigned after she had joined the Women's Auxiliary Air Force (WAAF). Apparently, she caught his eye when he issued her an order of some description and she told him to piss off. Stan liked women with a bit of spirit; he wasn't used to being argued with. Just how much spirit Olive had might have surprised him, if he'd known.

They tied the knot one stormy night in Central Otago and bought a property at Paremata, which in those days was just a little fishing village north of the somewhat larger fishing village of Wellington. It was where we four children — in descending order: Richard, me, Andrew and Elizabeth — were brought up.

It was an awesome place to be a kid; a massive harbour with endless mudflats surrounded by farms with high hills and lots of bush. It was a bit of a rough place in those days; no one had a lot of money, but in reflection it was paradise for a kid who loved adventure. If we weren't at school, my friends and I would be off before dawn fishing in the harbour or playing games like hide-and-seek in the hills. Mum and Dad didn't seem to worry too much about where we were, even when we came back home late in the evening dog-tired and covered in scratches.

When we were growing up, I think I knew my parents were a slightly odd couple. Stan seemed to be too old to be a dad; he was more a grandfather figure to us, really. While we wouldn't expect him to stand on the sidelines at the rugby in driving rain in the middle of winter, he was always full of great stories amassed from his very colourful career.

Stan joined the Royal Flying Corps as a boy apprentice in 1913, and after the First World War became a career soldier with the then newly formed Royal Air Force (RAF). Between wars he was stationed overseas in all manner of interesting locations, including the Middle East. Between 1926 and 1928 he was even based out the back in British India where one of his messmates stood out as a bit of a swashbuckler and went by the name of T. E. Shaw. Dad and the rest of the crew knew his real name, of course, was T. E. Lawrence or the more widely known 'Lawrence of Arabia'.

The stories! Stan reckoned when he was stationed in Iraq, he and his messmates used to keep a boot by their pillows so that when a tarantula wandered in the door (as they often did), someone would yell 'Tarantula up!' and the poor critter would die in a hail of boot leather.

On the airfields, it was common for the ground crew to carry pistols, so that if a pilot messed up and his kite caught fire, he was quickly put out of his misery rather than be left to burn to death.

'Did you ever see that happen?' we would ask, wide-eyed.

'Ho yes,' Stan would reply.

'Oooooh,' we'd go.

Dad was a bit of a disciplinarian, but let's face it, he had his work cut out for him with four very spirited kids and an equally spirited young wife. I reckon we all kept him young. Stan had to work like a dog to provide for his young family; he certainly wasn't afraid of it.

'Work hard,' he used to tell us solemnly, 'and doors will open.'

I've never forgotten that piece of wisdom.

=

Mum was at least as colourful as Stan. To buck social trends back then by marrying a man twice her age was brave, but you could never accuse Granny Olive (as everyone knew her once our kids were born) of lacking the courage of her convictions. She was born in Ngahere, on the southern banks of the Grey River, on the West Coast of the South Island, before moving upriver to Ahaura and then on to Central Otago.

Olive grew up with a love of the outdoors and was a very accomplished climber, knocking off many of New Zealand's highest peaks, including Malte Brun (3198 m) and Tititea/Mount Aspiring (3033 m), and almost bagged the highest — Aoraki/Mount Cook (3724 m) — on a number of occasions. The most significant peak she climbed, in my opinion, was Mount Hector in the Tararua Range, because she took me along and it was the first peak we climbed together. I must have been about 11 years old. We set off from Otaki Forks and I still remember coming over the first big hill and getting a full view of Maungahuka peak — it just looked so awesome and I have never forgotten the thrill I felt. The experience bonded me forever with the bush and the mountains and I have Granny Olive to thank for that.

※

It seems, looking back, that I knew the end of the golden weather had come the moment I first sat behind a desk at Paremata School. Some people are designed by the Big Guy in the Sky to love rules and regulations, but I wasn't one of them. It probably wouldn't have been so bad if I couldn't see the hills and the sky through the windows, but I could. My eyes constantly strayed there in the middle of the chaos and confusion that was my primary school education. I could see the birds flying around, smugly revelling in their freedom, and it felt cruel and unnatural that I had to be cooped up in class. When I went home and watched *Ivanhoe*, my favourite TV show, I felt full of sympathy for the swashbuckling knight, shackled hand and foot, languishing in the grim dungeons of Torquilstone Castle. Shit, that was school right there.

My soul rebelled. Most of my classmates seemed at home in the strictly controlled environment of the classroom, but fortunately my free-spirited young soul was not alone. I had a couple of hard-out mates like Brian King, Phillip Hague Smith and Billy Curtis, who were just as keen as I was to do a runner from school whenever the opportunity arose. Who knows how my teachers put up with me — professional pride, I suppose, if nothing else, but full credit to them anyway. It's not that I was incapable; I could swim, run fast and was smart enough to catch frogs, fish and possums. It's just that none of it was part of the school curriculum, and all the stuff that was — the stuff the teachers wrote on the blackboard — was like software written for a totally different operating system. I was fairly sure I was stupid, but I wasn't stupid enough to believe there was no value in an education. I knew you needed a certain amount of it to get the kind of job that would pay well enough to allow you to do the stuff that you really wanted to do, which was run, jump, swim, dive, hunt, fish and climb.

For a while, I fixed my hopes on my Bonus Bonds coming through, or striking it rich in the Golden Kiwi. But as time went by, hope faded. There seemed no getting away from the fact that I needed to achieve some actual learning. My teachers kept Granny Olive informed of my progress, or lack of it; in spite of it all, she reckoned there was a brain in there somewhere. When they suggested that I be held back a year, she told them off and was adamant that I was just as gifted as her other three children. I was touched by her faith, but sceptical. After all, mothers didn't have to have expertise in anything beyond cooking, cleaning and telling kids off, did they?

However, everything changed when a certain teacher, Mrs Thompson, came along and messed with my mind. She was 40-odd, I suppose, and rather lovely looking. Her husband earned good money, so she wasn't trying to get rich out of teaching. Mrs T was in it because she wanted to be, and that's why she took enough of an interest to help me discover learning, in spite of me.

It all began one lovely summer's day. My class was housed in the old Paremata chemist shop while a nice new classroom was being built for us at the school. Mrs T stood at the front of the room and we stared back at her like a mob of steers staring at a tractor. Her tone as she began speaking — nice as pie, friendly — should have alerted me straight away: I was pretty good at smelling a rat in those days. She said that she needed to divide the class into two groups for reading, because they didn't have enough books or something. The good readers (or 'brainy bastards' as I disdainfully called them) would be in Group A. The strugglers (or the 'dumb bastards', in whose number I proudly included myself) would make up Group B.

I received this news with nothing more than a mental shrug. In fact, I tuned out pretty much immediately, being much more preoccupied with glaring at one of my mates who had just used his favourite big Molly to smash me in marbles. I was hurting big time. That was much more significant than the kind of trifling administrative crap that teachers dreamed up in the deluded belief that it might change anything.

I dimly registered that Mrs T was still talking. She announced that each student would decide for themselves which group they belonged in. She said she felt confident we were all mature enough to make a fair assessment of our own abilities. And with that, for the first time in years of seeking it, Mrs T suddenly had my full attention.

'Just be honest with yourselves,' she said.

There was a buzz of whispered conversation and a few sniggers. Like me, everyone else had just worked out that — with a surname starting with 'B' for Baldwin — I was going to be the first in the hot seat to make a mature and honest decision about how shit-hot a reader I was. Christ! If I chose Group B then my best mates, who were equally as dumb as me, might choose Group A and I'd be stuck with a bunch of dumb people I didn't like. But if I chose Group A — yeah, right — my mates might choose Group B and I'd be stuck with a bunch of dorky, brainy bastards I didn't like.

With great relish Mrs T picked up her class roll book. She consulted it and fixed me with a predatory stare. She knew me well enough, and my reading level; she seemed to be having trouble controlling her expression.

'Well, Mr Baldwin,' she said sweetly. 'Which group do you think you'd like to be in?'

All eyes were upon me. Amongst the sea of smirking faces, I could see the delighted expectation lighting up the dials of my mates. I felt beads of sweat break out; the atmosphere in the room was electric. I opened my mouth and there was a creak of chairs as everyone leaned forward to hear what came out.

I swallowed hard and, on a mad impulse, blurted: 'Group A, please, Mrs T!'

My announcement was greeted with a brief, shocked pause before a gale of abandoned laughter rolled through the room. Some kids — my mates, most notably — were actually rolling around on the floor in hysterics. It was one of those rare moments in world history when a single event brings together a diverse group of people with widely varying religious, ethnic and socio-economic backgrounds to speak in one clear and united voice. If they had been able to draw sufficient breath, they would have chorused: 'David Baldwin is Group B material, but only because there is no Group Z!'

It took Mrs T a full 15 minutes to restore some semblance of order in the class, but she was in no rush. I could tell she was enjoying herself. I'd been tormenting teachers and kids alike for years and this was plainly payback. But the class was in for a second shock. Instead of reminding me that she was after my *honest* assessment of my reading abilities, Mrs T nodded serenely and said: 'Fair enough, Mr Baldwin. Group A it will be.'

Another 10 minutes of hilarity ensued.

In the final wash-up, Group A consisted of four brainy bastards and me. The remaining 25 students — including all of my good mates — opted for Group B. I fucked that one up, and my acute discomfort lasted throughout the first few sessions. The other four members of my reading group would each read an extract from Dr Seuss's *The Cat in the Hat* with all the gusto and expression of John frigging Gielgud's *Hamlet*, and then sit in silence as I stumbled in a dull monotone, cheeks flaming, from one mangled word to the next as my grubby index finger traced each line.

But two unexpected things happened. First, I had to modify my views on 'brainy bastards'. They didn't snigger or sigh at all as I blundered along: all four were patient and encouraging, which not only gave me confidence but also earned them my undying gratitude. And second, my reading improved at a rate that I would not have believed possible. Once the dust had settled and my mates began to realise that I was not going to be humiliated and dropped down from Group A to Group B, they began to treat me as though I was a card-carrying brainy bastard. It was all very confusing. It was also my first glimpse into the way peer-group pressure works. If you're amongst people who are convinced they're no-hopers, you don't have a hope; but if you're among people who want and expect to achieve and are prepared to work to do it, you're likely to get carried along for the ride.

Who knows whether I was the intended target of Mrs T's initiative, or whether there were others, too. The fact that she didn't tell me to get real when I first chose Group A suggests she thought she spied some sort of learning potential in there somewhere. At the time I resented her bitterly, but as the weeks went by I felt grudging admiration and this has only intensified down the years. Credit where it's due: I wouldn't be where I am now if not for Mrs T.

—

Richard and I were home alone, as we quite often were, when our lives changed dramatically. It was 1966 and I was nine. Richard happened to glance out the window and said: 'Shit. There's been an accident.' There was nothing particularly unusual about this. From our house we could see in the distance a notorious bend in the road where accidents were common. Joining Richard, I soon saw the tell-tale cluster of red flashing lights that indicated something serious.

'I'm going to have a look,' Richard said, pulling on his boots.

'I'm coming, too,' I said, but he told me to stay put. Arguing with big brothers didn't pay dividends in those days, so I shrugged and did what I was told.

He was back 10 minutes later, white as a ghost. 'It's Dad,' he said. 'Dad's had a crash. They're taking him to hospital.'

Stan was lucky to live. He ended up in Lower Hutt Hospital in full traction for weeks before spending six months rehabilitating at Silverstream Hospital. Even when he was released, Dad was physically never quite the same. It seems you can recover much more easily from major trauma when you're young, but he was old.

Things had been tight enough for us with Stan's income coming in, but now he was out of action we were in dire straits. There was no accident compensation scheme back then, and we were on our own. Andrew and Elizabeth were packed off to live with rellies, while Granny Olive worked as the school janitor and took on extra cleaning on the side. Richard and I helped, too. Sometimes we stuck around after school to help Mum clean or stoke the old coal boiler. Quite often Mum and I would shoot off before four o'clock in the morning with our two dogs, Ricky and Camellia, jumping and yipping with excitement beside us to do extra cleaning jobs like the Mana Cruising Club at Ngatitoa Domain. I didn't see it as a bad time.

YEARNING FOR FREEDOM

It gets pretty cold on the Kapiti Coast in winter, but we were OK. Richard and I shared a tiny room, and we had a dog each to cuddle up to on cold nights. Man, with two boys and two dogs in close confines, the room was savoury in the morning, but it was great. Another measure of how hard up we were is that once I went off to a mate's birthday party with a couple of boiled eggs as his present. I remember his mum showing me in, smiling at me and my gift, then excusing herself to go off down the hall and scream at my mother down the telephone. It all sort of passed me by at the time as I was more interested in ripping into the food and playing birthday games than sorting out what my mate's mum's problem was. The great thing about kids is they live very much in their own little world. It can take a lot to reach them.

My world mostly involved the stuff I got up to outside of school. As soon as the bell went I was gone, fishing or chasing rabbits. I was desperate to get a gun so I could hunt properly, but Olive wasn't having a bar of it. By doing odd jobs, I managed to save up the $45 I needed to buy a Marlin .22 rifle on the sly.

I hid it under my good mate Richard Peck's house. He and I would go off shooting, often heading out into the countryside on the unit train that ran between Palmerston North and Pukerua Bay with our rifles (you could do that in those days). We would return the same way with our rifles and a few dead bunnies; I would stash the gun back under Richard's house and then take the rabbits home. Olive was delighted with the free tucker, but obviously a bit suspicious.

'Where did these come from?' she would ask.

'Oh, a mate gave them to me,' I would reply breezily.

By now Olive had taken over the family finances, such as they were, from Stan. There was a nasty surprise waiting for her in there. She discovered that he was paying maintenance to another woman and another bunch of kids over in England, and when she confronted him with the discovery, she learned that there was yet another woman and child kicking about the landscape, too. It must have been a shock, and most people would probably have told Stan to get stuffed at that point. But Granny Olive was no ordinary woman; after she'd thought it all through she must have decided that, in the end, none of it made a difference to what she and Stan had. They were soulmates. When he was well enough to come out of hospital, she welcomed him back.

Even when Stan went back to work — he had to lie about his age to get a job — we were still hard up. It must have been an enormous sacrifice, with money so tight, but my parents managed to find the cash to send first Richard and then me off to board at Marlborough Boys' College over in Blenheim. They spoke of the school reverently, as though it had a tremendous reputation, but in reality it was a pretty rough outfit. Still, I made a new set of mates and had some pretty good times, and we got to see the big wide world outside of Paremata on our own for the first time. Richard and I only lasted a few years at Marlborough, due to our somewhat wayward and free-spirited antics and the fact that the family coffers were running dry. Time away from home meant that when we arrived back at Paremata and enrolled at local Tawa College to finish high school, we had developed a very independent, worldly view of life. Richard and I are both eternally grateful to our parents for that.

The last couple of years I spent at Tawa were great fun; all four of us Baldwin kids were together, and I loved the hard-out sport, which included First XV rugby and indoor basketball.

It also helped that I had worked out a method for getting all of my learning done. This new-found approach to study had seen me win the top student prize in my fourth form class at Marlborough. With all the will in the world, and all the help from well-meaning teachers and textbooks, my mind couldn't seem to absorb information in a normal way. So I learned to rewrite all of the information I was given by the teacher, along with textbook and handout material, into a special format that my brain could comprehend and which I then learned by rote. Mnemonics had a lot to do with it. Computer geeks would probably refer to this as some type of software synchronisation. I called this material 'Dave Speel' (it speaks volumes that this is how I spelled 'Spiel'), and it helped me upload all the information I needed so I could then flexibly apply it to answer any particular examination question relating to the subject I had studied. It was laborious — I spent twice as long over stuff as my classmates — but it seemed to work and I managed to get University Entrance. Mum was overjoyed!

Looking back, I have to say that it's not only about discovering your own learning style; it's also about having good, understanding teachers. It can make all the difference to a kid's chances of success. One teacher in particular, a certain Mrs Waugh, really made it happen for me in English. Not only was she inspirational, but her arm-twisting and encouragement to learn all about a Wilfred Owen poem describing the horrors of trench warfare in the First World War got me through School Certificate English. The science teachers I had unfortunately didn't have the same ability to captivate me and I ended up failing that subject — kind of ironic, given where my life's path has taken me. So I spent the rest of my time at college studying history and geography.

Meanwhile, I had upgraded from my rabbit gun to something capable of taking down bigger game. Ex-Army Lee-Enfield and M1 .303 rifles were plentiful in those days: when I was 15, I bought a Short Magazine Lee-Enfield (SMLE) cut down from its fully-wooded military configuration. I got it for $35 from Tisdalls.

Boy oh boy, what a cannon! It fired off 150-grain lead-headed rounds with a deafening roar. Once I had my hands on this little beauty, I headed off into the bush as soon as I could to 'get me a stag'. It's amazing how loose the world was then, as no one seemed too fussed about me and one of my buddies at the time, Geoffrey Childs, heading off into the mountains by ourselves with only the most basic gear. We entered the Tararuas via Levin and did the long, arduous climb up onto Arete, where we got stuck in a tiny New Zealand Forest Service bivvy for two days in a storm. On the third morning the weather cleared so we headed off in different directions to hunt alone. Geoff headed north and I headed south, but we hadn't been apart for more than 15 minutes when I happened to stop to wipe the sweat from my eyes and saw a stag standing, perfectly still, on the skyline above me on the exact top of Arete. Till the day I die I will never forget the thrill of my first sight of a mighty stag alone in the mountains.

After a moment or two, the stag swung its head and disappeared from view. I charged up the hillside to the ridge, my heart thumping in my chest, and cautiously advanced over the crest. There he was, only 50 yards or so from my vantage point, chewing on a bit of mountain grass. With trembling hands, I quietly chambered a round and took aim. I didn't even know which of the pinholes in the aperture sights I was meant to use to line him up, but the range was so close it hardly mattered. I squeezed the trigger and the report echoed around the hills. The animal staggered.

I fired off another five rounds in quick succession, methodically working my way around each of the various pinholes located in the gunsight just to be sure I used the right one. It was a great relief when the stag eventually fell down in a heap.

By the time I reached him, the stag — my first — was dead, the light of the early morning sky reflecting in his big, wet, unseeing eye. I was grinning like a madman, and I sat down on his warm chest and basked in the moment. It turned out he'd been part of a small herd of deer and his five mates were running down to the safety of the bush below. Deer are a sight to behold at full gallop.

It's funny how certain memorable pictures can stick in one's mind. I can clearly remember, as I sat on my first lavishly perforated and very dead stag, the panoramic view up there from Arete; of the Manawatu Plains, including Lake Horowhenua, the Foxton coastline and Palmerston North. I had no idea at that time that this area was to be my future. I had realised my dream of successfully stalking my first deer. And it was the beginning of another: to spend as much of the rest of my life as I could out in places like this, doing what I was doing.

Maybe one day, when I've passed over, I'll have to look that stag in the eye (I can't imagine a heaven without deer).

'Sorry, mate,' I'll say to him. 'No hard feelings, bro. I had to do what I had to do.'

I hope he'll understand.

CHAPTER 2

TIME TO GET ME SOME SCHOOLING

Since I had a piece of paper entitling me to go to university, it seemed logical that I should do just that in 1975. As the Monty Python Sergeant Major screams to a platoon of young soldiers in their famous parade skit, 'Today we're going to do marching up and down the square. That is unless any of you have got something better to do?'

Granny Olive was determined that I should do it. She had ended her own formal education at the completion of Form 2 (Year 8 in today's money), like many women of her generation. I had no real idea what I wanted to do, but I thought something that got me into the great outdoors would be about right. I didn't want to be a farmer, and they didn't have all those dream degrees in parks and recreation and tourism and outdoor adventure guiding that they do now. So I decided to have a crack at surveying, and duly enrolled in the intermediate year at Victoria University of Wellington.

I quickly worked out that it was all a gigantic mistake. I wasn't really in any mood to study; I found the lecture theatres at Victoria very claustrophobic and I simply didn't fit in with all the urban brainy bastards. It just wasn't me. Likewise, the life of a surveyor sounded great, but maths and physics were never my strong suit, and here I was trying to pretend I was interested in a heavily maths-based discipline.

Nor did I have much of a social life. I went to plenty of parties, and I mostly enjoyed myself, but I didn't have any luck with women. They laughed at my jokes and all the rest, but when push came to shove they seemed to regard me as a bit loud, a bit of a show-off.

Fair enough, I thought.

Looking back, the highlight of my university day back then was sitting in the library and ogling the Southern Tararuas and Mount Hector out the window and across the harbour. I pined for the hills.

On one of those occasions, I was reading the *Dominion* newspaper and spied an advertisement for a driver to do delivery work around Wellington.

Hmmm, I thought. Hmmmmmmmm, I thought some more.

I looked up from the newspaper to the Tararuas with an ache in my heart.

I didn't know what I was doing in that bloody place so I sprang into action and a minute later I had contacted the boss. Five minutes later, I had jacked up an interview. Fifty-five minutes later, I was presenting myself to Skellerup at their head office. Fifty-eight minutes later, I was all signed up as their new distribution executive (or delivery boy, in the rather demeaning patois of the day).

I had gone from feeling run down and low to exhilarated within a single hour; I felt as if a weight had been lifted off my shoulders. I was free!

I sometimes wonder whether the books and papers I left on the desk in the university library are still there. I never went back to check.

Granny Olive, needless to say, was devastated. Every time she looked at me, her face collapsed into an expression of purest misery. She just couldn't understand how I could thumb my nose at this great opportunity for free higher education that she had been denied. But after all those years spent shackled hand and foot in the grim dungeons of Torquilstone Castle, I wasn't inclined to listen to her tearful pleas to reconsider. I was free, and I vowed that, henceforth, I would forever abstain from any literature or schooling. I'd had a gutsful of the classroom.

—

While I was driving for Skellerup, I moonlighted as a 'sanitation facility hygiene executive', cleaning 24 floors of male toilets in a big skyscraper on The Terrace in Wellington. I genuinely loved the job and used to whistle while I worked. The great thing about dunny cleaning is that not only are you indispensable, but they can't demote you to a position any lower on the food chain.

There is a certain power. One night some big shot hurried into a toilet I had just cleaned and banged the door. Disturbed by the noises coming from the cubicle, I did a quick inspection after he came out. He'd shat all over the place, even up the wall. I gave him a right old bollocking in not-so-Queen's English. You could tell he wasn't used to being yelled at, and he went to slink guiltily off. He sped up noticeably when I told him I was going to rub his nose in it as I did when house-training our dog!

After driving for Skellerup, I had a succession of other menial jobs — farm work for Mr Clements in Pukerua Bay, possuming, roof tiling for Monier — and spent all my spare time hunting in the Tararuas. Poor old Granny Olive was torn; while she was afraid I was becoming a waster, she was openly impressed with the money I was earning and only too happy to come along with me on my hunting trips.

I noticed, in particular, that she used to scale down her howling over my future as the roar — the best time for stag hunting — approached. I was happy to ask her along; she was great company with an encyclopaedic knowledge of native flora and fauna, and a superb bush cook to boot. Her favourite bit of the deer carcass was the heart, and whenever I brought one into the camp she'd squeal with delight and start joyfully yodelling for the next five minutes. As soon as we were back in town and there were no hunting expeditions in prospect, the tears, the sighing and the wringing of hands over the way I was squandering my many advantages would start up all over again.

TIME TO GET ME SOME SCHOOLING

One of the most memorable hunts we went on during these years was the roar of 1977, when Dave Roberts, Mum and I walked to the Elder Bivvy on the Renata Ridge to get us a big stag.

After a good overnight snooze, Dave headed off with his dog Hercules in one direction while Mum and I and our dog Camellia made a beeline for a valley running off Mount Aston where I'd had some luck hunting previously. We found a good spot in some ferns halfway up the mountainside and sat down. I used a rusty old pear tin I often carried on such trips to simulate a roar. Granny Olive was just opening her mouth to tell me I sounded like a constipated ram when there was an answering roar from quite close by. We both got a big shock. Mum told me later that it was the first time she'd heard a stag roar, and she reckoned he sounded as though he were constipated too!

Granny Olive had the binoculars, and she glassed the bushline.

'See anything?' I whispered.

'Not sure,' she breathed. 'But there's a funny-looking log sticking out over there...'

I grabbed the binos and had a look where she was indicating, a small outcrop of rocks in a steep tributary gully.

'It's a fucking stag!' I whispered.

'Language!' she hissed, but she was just as excited as I was.

I lay down and drew careful aim. It was 400 metres. I fired — and the stag stayed right where it was. I peered at it through my scope, wondering if it was a log, after all.

No, surely it was a stag. I fired again, with no visible effect.

'I'll have to go closer,' I told her, and made my way stealthily across the gully. When I was 50 metres from the beast, I lined him up again. It was a stag, all right, and obligingly, he was still no more than a metre away from where he'd been when I had my first crack at him. I settled the cross hairs just behind his shoulder and fired again. This time, I bowled him over.

There was a scuffling noise; Granny Olive appeared at my elbow, breathing heavily, her eyes shining.

'You got him!' she said.

We picked our way up to where the stag was lying. He had three bullet wounds, one of them in his hindquarters, and my guess is that this shot passed through both hip joints, locking them up. He couldn't do anything from that point on but wait for Big Old Daddy Dave to come and finish him off.

Back at the bivvy that evening, I solemnly promoted Mum from shooter's cook to shooter's mate. She was delighted, but it didn't stop her wailing and gnashing her teeth once we got back to town.

Slowly but surely her howling began to pay off, probably because I knew, deep down, that to have the lifestyle I really wanted, I would need some kind of 'ticket'. Most of my mates were well on the way to some sort of career certainty, with trade qualifications or degrees or diplomas of some description. Even I could see I was losing ground; doing bum jobs for other people was never going to get me into the position I wanted to be in (and I still hadn't collected on the Golden Kiwi).

So in 1977, I swallowed my pride and my misgivings and told Granny Olive that I would give academia another go. I thought that would keep her happy, so I felt a little put out when she burst into tears. However, they were tears of joy; she hugged me and promised that if I got a degree she would be happy with whatever I decided to do with my time after that, even if I chose to be a professional deer culler.

I presented myself at the enrolments advice desk at Massey University in Palmerston North. It was manned by a kindly old man by the name of Professor Mumford.

'So, what are you interested in studying?' he asked.

'I'm keen to do science,' I told him, 'but I'm not very good at it. So make it the easiest science degree you can work out, preferably without much science in it!'

He winked. 'Why, you've come to the right place,' he said, with a wry old smile.

Professor Mumford sorted me out with a set of papers that he thought would do the trick. Aghast, I realised he'd lined me up with a full portfolio of chemistry papers of one sort or another — chemistry, organic chemistry, biochemistry . . . Jeez, I couldn't even spell their long names, let alone guess what they were all about. I finished enrolment day with a sense of mounting dread of the study ahead and deep admiration for the professor's sales skills.

I sorted out a hostel room on campus and packed my few possessions (my rifle taking pride of place, of course) and prepared to set off. Granny Olive was radiantly happy, but when I met Camellia's eye, I saw my own miserable expression mirrored on her pissed-off little face. She seemed to know that the happy time she'd lately spent gallivanting around in the bush was coming to an end, and I felt exactly the same.

To my shock, though, I really enjoyed myself. The lectures and labs weren't exactly the place to get an adrenalin buzz, and

I did it much harder than most of my classmates. I still had to convert all of the information we received in lectures and from textbooks into 'Dave Speel' in order to get my head around it. The compensations, though, included the beautiful campus at Massey and, of course, access to the university's legendary social life, which centred around the Fitzherbert Hotel, or the Fitz, as it is fondly (if pretty dimly) remembered by Massey alumni everywhere.

And things only got better in the second half of the year, when I got my hostel room to myself. I'd had six different roommates in four months and eventually no one seemed to want to hole up with me at all. I don't know whether it was me — coming in at odd hours in my tiny green hunting shorts and bloodstained bush shirt, carrying my rifle and grinning through my tangled hair and bushy beard — or whether it was them. In the end, I didn't much care. I had my big double room to myself.

The fact that I was happy in my work was reflected in my academic performance, too, and I found that I was actually footing it. I was rubbing shoulders with people who desperately wanted good marks because they were intent on going to vet school or med school (you could do the Medical Intermediate outside of the medical colleges in those days), and it was quite a competitive environment. We were all conscious that everyone was watching everyone else, and trying to work out where each person ranked. To my surprise, people even seemed to be keeping an eye on me. This seemed ridiculous, until one day — a real turning point in the way I thought about myself — when a mate of mine asked me what I was going to do when I graduated. Even the 'when' gave me a little thrill. I put on the straightest face I could manage and said: 'I reckon I'll be a doctor.' I glared at him, daring him to laugh.

Not the slightest trace of amusement crossed his face, and he nodded seriously.

Bugger me, I thought. He actually thinks I can do it.

Self-confidence counts for so much and after that little conversation I decided, yup, by hook or by crook I was going to be a doctor of medicine! Bring it on, baby!

At the end of my first year at Massey I passed all eight papers and got a B+ average. This wasn't good enough to get into medical school, but it didn't matter. I knew I could do better and I now had the confidence to kick arse and get a good science degree that would hopefully gain me entry into Otago Medical School at New Zealand's oldest university.

=

In the summer break, I managed to wangle a job with the New Zealand Forest Service doing deer surveys in Mount Aspiring National Park. This meant spending most of the time in the mountains and valleys with a team of three other blokes collecting information on how many deer were about. The Powers That Be could have just asked the local hunters, but ah, well . . . It was a great job, and the fact that I was hidden away in the Southern Alps meant I could save a lot of money for my next year at Massey. I was in the company of some good bastards, too. There was the odd flare-up, of course: the discomforts and inconveniences of living with a bunch of other strong-willed men for extended periods of time made it inevitable that there would be differences of opinion. But fights amongst men are different to the kinds of fights women have. Men settle things in a quick, glorious blaze, like a bushfire, whereas women tend to let ill feeling smoulder away underground, like a peat fire.

One bloke I couldn't get over was Terry. He was a pretty unassuming-looking character, a bit rough in many ways, but he seemed to exert some sort of mysterious power over women. His exploits were legendary, and unusually in these situations, it wasn't just him who said so. One day, I sadly told him about my inability to get beyond first base with women.

'Nothing to it, Dave,' he said, and beckoned me to lean in closer. 'What you've got to do when you're interested in a woman is show her you're keen, and then back right off. Trust me. It works!'

I was sceptical, but filed the information away for future reference.

The second year of my science degree began with a hiss and a roar. I was all fired up to kick arse and get this thing over with. An old mate's grandmother wanted a boarder so I took up the opportunity to hole up with her rather than go flatting. I hated cooking, and she so badly needed someone to fatten up that I figured I was doing her a favour. And (no disrespect to Granny Peterson) her lifestyle wasn't going to distract me from my studies.

Sadly (as it seemed at the time), Granny Petersen announced

she had to leave Palmy just after mid-year, so I got the boot and had to go looking for a flat after all. I found a place with three others: Possum, Dot and Sandi. Possum and Dot thought I would be a good flatmate but Sandi was sceptical, as she thought I was a bit of a dick. But Sandi was outvoted and I got a room.

Sandi needn't have worried. None of my flatmates saw much of me for the rest of the year because I worked like a dog; I was on a mission to get my damned degree over. The only break I had in my routine was Thursday night, which was my night for cooking. I perfected a massive beef stew that practically cooked itself and dished it out like clockwork every Thursday. I would bolt mine down and get right back to studying.

Towards the end of the year I started to notice my washing being folded and things seeming a bit tidier around my room. Either little naked men were responsible, or it was someone in the flat. Possum didn't like housework, and Dot wasn't overly domesticated, so it had to be Sandi. This was strange. I got the sense that Sandi might actually like me, so I decided to deploy the wisdom of Terry the Bushman. I showed a bit of interest and then went back to my books. It worked a treat; Sandi discovered that far from being a bit of a dick (or perhaps in spite of being a bit of a dick), I was actually her soulmate. Lucky is I!

We went out and hit it off really well. So well, in fact, that three days later I popped the question and I got the big 'YES'. Some things are just meant to be, I reckon, and it turned out Sandi agreed.

Soon after that, the academic year ended and I had a string of A passes — I was creaming it, and I only had one year to go. I did another three months in the bush with the Forest Service to save money, but it was different in the bush this time, because I just wanted to be doing things with Sandi. At least I got to meet some great people — people like Pete Devane, Bill Fluery and Stu McLaughlin, who have remained great mates.

===

In 1979, a good mate jacked Sandi and me up with a little flat in Palmerston North. We both worked very hard and the following October Sandi finished her BA and I graduated with a BSc majoring in biochemistry. Not only that, but my marks were good enough for admission to Otago Medical School. Sandi applied and got into Dunedin Teachers' College — we were made! Of course Granny Olive took full credit for my success and, I had to admit, without her expert application of every dark art in the emotional blackmailer's handbook, I wouldn't have been where I was (or indeed where I am now).

The following year, Sandi and I loaded up her little Honda Civic and headed off for Dunedin. We got a great little flat that overlooked the harbour and we soon settled into a routine with, as usual, lots of hard work. I was very fortunate; all I had to do was study, study and study, because Sandi took amazing care of me otherwise.

And study, study and study was what I *had* to do. It dawned on me soon after my first day at med school that I was staring down the nightmarish barrel of a further five years in the classroom in order to complete my degree. I was still a rote learner, which meant long hours of hard work converting the material I had been given each day into my 'Dave Speel'. There was also no real point in thinking about the future: I had to qualify in medicine before I could start thinking about what branch of medicine I would like to practise. So I just had to put my head down and tail up to get through it all. I felt not so much like a bird with clipped wings as a bird with no wings at all. Like Johnny Cash sang: I was doing my time and time kept marching on.

I did manage to get out for the odd bit of hunting. One day I hightailed it north to the Hampden State Forest looking for a nice fat deer to shoot. During my wanderings I came upon a big wild boar rooting around in the undergrowth without a care in the world. I'm no pig hunter but I will shoot one if I trip over it, so without further ado I sent a .222-calibre projectile through the boar's big, hairy chest.

Things didn't exactly go to plan. The pig swung its head towards me and glared at me with those mean, red piggy eyes, apparently completely unfazed by the bullet wound. As I watched through my telescopic sight, the beast started getting bigger and bigger. Since I wasn't fiddling with the magnification, that could mean only one thing.

I slammed another round up the spout as old piggy rumbled vengefully towards me. I steadied myself and fired, and it was with great relief that I saw it tumble over and lie still.

This whole experience only served to confirm me as a hunter of deer; those nice, gentle-eyed animals with a shy, retiring disposition, armed with nothing scarier than antlers and a mouthful of molars. I had a whole new respect for pig hunters and just how tough they have to be — facing a really pissed-off boar by yourself out in the bush has got to be dodgy.

Even people born to study — you know who you are, you smart-arsed bastards — find med school a hard slog. The rest of us need the occasional morale booster to keep us going; some kind of incentive or, at the very least, reassurance that it's all worthwhile. Near the end of my own exhausting journey a ray of hope came my way, in the unlikely form of a medical conference.

Even those who are born to plant kisses on the arses of others — you know who *you* are, too — struggle to enjoy conferences. The presentations are no different to lectures, really, except for the dispiriting knowledge that sitting through them isn't going to get you any closer to a degree. I generally spent them staring out the window or diligently doodling pictures on the refill pad that the drug companies thoughtfully provided. I drew aircraft, rifles and stags with improbably large sets of antlers. But the lectures were fun compared with the schmoozing that went on between sessions. The only way I coped with this part of the proceedings was to treat the whole thing as a kind of anthropological exercise.

David Attenborough's voice would start up in my head: 'And now, in the foyer outside the lecture theatre, we're privileged to watch one of the most intriguing rituals in nature, the kissing of the arse of the senior consultants and professorial staff. There now. See how the consultant holds court in the middle of a throng of white-coated inferiors. Every pronouncement is greeted with a range of exaggerated signals and overstated gestures of approval — hoots of laughter, wide grimaces of mirth, the vigorous nodding or shaking of heads. Every now and then, two consultants or professors will square off and exchange highly coded pleasantries, or engage in big-noting one-upmanship, the whole display attended appreciatively by their lessers, who watch tirelessly from the sideline for any opportunity to chip in with a witticism or observation that will mark them out from the crowd and brighten their career prospects. And there, outside the inner circle and recognisable by their lack of white coats, the outcasts stand awkwardly, waiting for any chance to catch a senior colleague's eye, maybe even a nod, or any sign of recognition of their existence. These are the medical students, the lowest of the low in this strictly hierarchical society, and they are, of course, resolutely ignored . . .'

At one of these excruciating events in my sixth year, when the end of my student days was so close I could almost taste it, I was trudging down the stairs into just such a throng looking for someone of my own status who might deign to chat to me. I couldn't see anyone I knew in the coatless outer ring, but I did spy a dishevelled old bloke in the corner who was keeping himself to himself. He looked like he might have been the cleaner so, being an ex-dunny cleaner myself, I wandered over to keep him company.

'Where do you work and what do you do?' I asked, as recommended by those who told us to treat these occasions as opportunities to make connections and soak up career advice.

'I spend all day sailing my boat around the Sounds,' he smiled. 'Otherwise, I do beggar all.'

I stared at him.

'I'm a GP,' he said, as though that explained it. 'Jacobsen's the name.' We shook hands, and I set about trying to find out if he was serious.

'Oh, yes,' he said. 'I only became a doctor so I could go sailing whenever I wanted to.'

It turned out that Dr Jacobsen was based in the small town of Havelock located in the Marlborough Sounds. He talked a little about general practice, but mostly he talked about his boat — a modified whale-chasing schooner — that he used to trip around the Sounds, do a bit of fishing and tend to the occasional house call en route.

'The rum flows freely at the end of the day!' he grinned.

I grinned back. It struck me that this slightly disreputable-looking man was the living, breathing vindication of my whole mission at med school! I said goodbye to Dr Jacobsen and went back to my studies with a fresh (or, more accurately, a new) enthusiasm. Perhaps it really was possible to fit employment around the lifestyle of your dreams.

―

A few months later, I got another boost to my morale in the shape of the 'elective' that sixth-year medical students are obliged to do. For three months, you get to choose where in New Zealand or overseas you'd like to travel, and in what branch of medicine you'd like to gain some experience. And it's all paid for.

Most of my medical student mates wasted no time in heading off to exotic places such as the New Hebrides (Vanuatu, these days), the Sudan or Namibia. I decided to divide my time. For the first six weeks I followed a forensic pathologist around as he did what pathologists do in the dingy old Wellington morgue.

TIME TO GET ME SOME SCHOOLING

I figured I'd save on suntan lotion, at least. Even though I hadn't been expecting a barrel of laughs, my first day was pretty sobering.

The pathologist met me and ushered me into the morgue.

'Our customers,' he said. 'One good thing: they don't talk back.'

There was a row of evenly spaced stainless-steel benches under harsh overhead lighting; the first six of these were occupied by dead bodies, each laid out neatly and as naked as they had come into the world.

'Unexplained deaths,' the pathologist said. 'It's our job to do a full post-mortem on each of them to find out the cause of death.'

I had seen dead bodies before, of course. Quite apart from the hundreds of different animals I had personally dispatched and butchered, I had seen a post-mortem performed in the second year of my training, and throughout my degree we had done quite a bit of work with human cadavers. But post-mortems have a way of underlining the facts of life and death like nothing else. In the hands of a skilled pathologist, it takes only a matter of minutes for a human body — a miraculous machine that takes years to develop and grow — to be reduced to a carcass and a few little tubs of offal. Each organ is thoroughly inspected, weighed and then chopped up into smaller bits for microscopic analysis. It's quite freaky to watch.

Throughout the first couple of autopsies, the pathologists were watching me to see if I was going to turn green, keel over or anything entertaining like that. But I wasn't bothered — or at least, my discomfort was more existential than physical. Everyone knows on a theoretical level that their body contains organs such as a heart, lungs, liver and intestines. But it's quite another thing to see them removed from an ordinary-looking body, to get intimately acquainted with their individual texture, the heft of them, even their smell.

The brain fascinated me most. You use a little circular saw to cut around the skull; the top part is lifted off to reveal something like a wrinkly old sea sponge, quivering there in its anatomically correct position. Every time I looked at a brain, I found it hard to believe that someone's entire world had existed in such a nondescript blob of jelly — all their thoughts, memories, their personality and their intelligence. It gave me a huge respect for the human body, but it also impressed on me the notion that for all its incredible complexity, our body is just a machine in the end, like a car. But unlike a car, you only get one, and you've got to look after it properly. Once you've crashed it, or allowed it to fall apart through poor maintenance, that's it. You don't get another.

I spent the second six weeks of my elective at Taupo Medical Centre. Doctors Tangi Martin, John de van Taylor and the new doc in town, Pete Battersby, who became a lifelong friend of mine, were all good Kiwi jokers. Taupo was a bit of a backwater in those days, so the practice had a rural flavour and lots of the varied work that made each day interesting and no two days the same. Forestry was a key industry in the district. If ignorance of good health and safety practice is bliss, then your average Taupo forestry worker was pretty bloody happy. From a personal perspective, this was an excellent state of affairs as I was keen to get a bit of experience suturing wounds. There's nothing like a big chainsaw wound to keep a young medical student and his needle and catgut happily occupied for hours. Most of the workers we saw didn't use the protective mail trousers that OSH insists upon these days, so we tended to see lots of cuts to the front of the upper legs. Those big saws can kick back viciously, and if you're not wearing a hard hat then you're quite likely to sustain a bad facial or head wound. Others managed to cut their hands badly, too. All in all, I got the kind of experience you don't often get outside a war zone.

Dealing with farmers and forestry workers most of the time meant there were very few airs and graces about the Taupo Medical Centre — everyone called a spade a spade. It was a breath of fresh air for someone who despised the Great Chain of Being at med school, but it could come as a bit of a shock to those who were at home in that world.

One day a bloke presented himself to Dr Tangi as the short-term locum the practice was seeking. I could tell Tangi didn't like this fella as soon as he walked in — something to do with his three-piece suit, perhaps, or his overdone aftershave. Dr Tangi's expression darkened further as Dr Fancy Pants introduced himself, casually dropping the name of the prestigious university at which he'd studied and handing over a hefty CV, assuring Dr Tangi that all of the many scientific papers he'd published in peer-reviewed journals were there, along with . . .

'Don't show me all this shit,' said Tangi. 'Where's your practising certificate?'

Dr Fancy Pants turned pale, rummaged in his suit pocket and passed him the little piece of paper that confirmed he was certified to practise medicine in New Zealand.

Tangi glanced at it and said: 'Fine. Now, piss off and do some work.' Without further ado, he turned around and headed home for lunch. I swear the locum stood there for five minutes holding his huge CV, clearly contemplating his unaccustomed low place in the food chain at Taupo Medical Centre. I left him to it.

My six weeks in Taupo whizzed past, and when they came to an end, so did eight straight years of university training. So, in 1984 I was handed the piece of paper that confirmed I had graduated MBChB — *Medicinae Baccalaureus, Baccalaureus Chirurgiae* — which I understand is Latin for 'Medical Brainy Bastard'.

I was quite rightly very proud and excited about this, not only because it had all seemed so highly improbable only a decade or so ago (and even now, I have to pinch myself), but also because it meant I could get on with the real part of my life armed with some actual earning potential. My excitement was nothing compared to the pride I saw in Sandi's face. She had supported me both financially and psychologically ever since we met, and I'm sure she felt my success was 'our success' and just reward for her sacrifices as much as my hard work. And if Sandi and I were pleased, Mum was positively over the moon. My very gleeful mother spent the next few months crowing about me to her poor browbeaten relatives and friends on the phone. She was adamant that she could have done the same had she not been so poor and downtrodden as a kid. I bet they would have given anything for caller ID back in those days!

But anyway, what the hell . . . I was rapt! I had certainly come a long way from being a wayward, free-spirited deer hunter in those turbulent teenage years to being a respectable doctor and hubby.

CHAPTER 3

I CULD NOT SPEL DOKTA BUT NOW I ARE ONE

The end of my formal medical training signalled the beginning of my real medical training, which, some would argue, continues to this day. Newly qualified doctors are entitled to wear a nice, shiny name badge with, say, 'Dr Dave Baldwin' emblazoned on it, but it would take a special sort of personality to believe that's all that is needed to go out there and do no harm. The profession is regrettably full of such personalities — you know who you are — but I am not one of them.

When the moment came for me to pin my badge on for my first day at work as a house surgeon at the orthopaedic department of

Hutt Hospital, I had to have several goes at it; not because I lack fine motor skills, you understand, but because I was pretty sure the label didn't fairly represent the contents.

Christ, I thought. What if someone asks me a question? You know, the kind of question doctors are supposed to know the answer to?

It took a little while to feel at ease. It helped that a mate of mine, Chris Williams, had been assigned to Hutt too, so we could both feel like dicks together.

I first met Chris in 1980 over my dead body. On your first day at Otago Medical School, you all creep into the Anatomy Dissection Facility where each student is assigned a cadaver to dissect. Each of these bodies is donated by its very kind former owner in the interests of science. The hope is that by cutting them up, the students gain a good practical knowledge of human anatomy that will stand them in good stead throughout their careers, which in turn benefits humanity. Chris and I were allocated the same body on our first day.

We got to know each other pretty well over the next few months. Right from the start, I had Chris pegged for a perfectionist; it showed as much in the way he dissected out the musculocutaneous nerve of the arm as in how he combed his hair. I've been called lots of things in my time, but never a perfectionist, so this little personality trait of Chris's ensured we were going to clash.

Sure enough, one fine day after Chris had spent hours dissecting out some fancy nerve deep in our body's arm, he headed off for a break, a coffee and a pie. I waved to him as I arrived at the facility. When I addressed our body, I was fascinated by Chris's work, but damn it all, I thought. Why not dig a little deeper? He won't mind.

It got really interesting as I burrowed away in this half-dissected arm. I just carried on following various stringy bits and pieces, with huge names that I couldn't pronounce, all the way down to the bone. I learned a lot on the way, but when I compared what the arm looked like when Chris had finished with it and what it looked like now, I had to admit that my dissection technique was a little bit looser than his.

Just as I was pondering what to do, Chris wandered back in, all coffeed up and happy, until he spied the end result of my additional work to his fine dissection. He went all pale and po-faced and I felt suddenly deeply unwanted.

I decided it was best if I shot through while he was still in the speechless stage of his grief. He didn't talk to me for a few months afterwards, but it's funny how things turn out . . . His finicky dissection technique is why he has ended up a top orthopaedic surgeon, while I'm still more of the butcher type, but what's harder to explain is how we ended up best mates. I was even best man at his wedding. I suppose opposites attract.

Orthopaedics is, crudely speaking, the science of fixing bones and joints. Most of the patients in the ward at Hutt Hospital were there for elective surgery (that is, pre-planned as opposed to acute or emergency surgery), and I soon got used to the ward routine of clocking patients in pre-surgery and then discharging them after they'd had a taste of the orthopaedic surgeon's knife (or the drill and chainsaw in the case of bone surgery). There was nothing much to this: it involved running through a checklist with the patient to make sure everything was working as expected and ensuring they knew how to care for their wounds and injuries.

The remainder of the patients in the ward were recovering from broken bones they had received during accidents. Most were elderly people who had slipped or tripped over and broken hips and stuff, but there were younger people (motorcyclists were over-represented in this group) who'd broken bones as well, most commonly femurs (thigh bones) and arm bones.

Then there were the more minor injuries, such as dislocated shoulders or run-of-the-mill wrist and ankle fractures, which were dealt with at the orthopaedic outpatient clinic. As the official orthopaedic house surgeons, it fell to Chris and me to attend to these. We were both pretty keen to gain experience in setting broken bones; sometimes patients would watch, bemused, as two fresh-faced young doctors jockeyed to be the one who attended to them, especially if it was a dislocated shoulder.

We both loved relocating shoulders. This was achieved using a manipulation technique known as Kocher's manoeuvre, where you bend the patient's affected arm at the elbow, rotate it to the side until you feel resistance, then rotate it forwards again, whereupon the ball of the arm joint will slip back into its socket with a satisfying and very audible 'clunk'. Maybe it was the clunk, or maybe it was the instant relief from the pain of dislocation that it offered the patient, but both Chris and I became obsessed with getting in first on these, to the point where I actually bribed an accident and emergency clerk with chocolate to send any patients my way that presented in the fracture room with shoulder dislocations.

This paid big dividends when — perhaps because there was ice on the footpaths or there was a skateboarding tournament on somewhere nearby — three dislocated shoulders came in one glorious day, one after another. Chris was distraught when he found out. To add insult to injury, he was also obliged to complete the paperwork that described my skill and prowess. He was even more upset when he learned about the underhand tactics I had used to get the jump on him. But he soon found ways of getting even. By the time we'd finished at the orthopaedic department, we'd done roughly equal numbers of Kocher's manoeuvres.

The lot of the house surgeon — the fancy name for an apprentice doctor, really — is to be rotated through various departments of a hospital in what are known as 'runs'. During the two years I spent at Hutt Hospital, I did runs in orthopaedics, general medicine, surgery, paediatrics (fixing kids) and obstetrics (attending women in childbirth). I also did a run in psychiatry over at the mental hospital at Porirua.

I enjoyed all of them, and I knew I was acquiring some amazing experience. Hutt Hospital just rocked for me; the culture there was very supportive and wholly focused on getting the job done, and it wasn't a huge hospital with a large medical staff, so you got to know everyone and they got to know you. Best of all, there was none of the hierarchical bullshit that you seem to get everywhere else in the profession: most of the holier-than-thou academic wankers were stationed across the harbour in Wellington Hospital, and they left us alone.

Because of the very long hours (sometimes over 120 hours a week if we spent a weekend on call) I gained a huge amount of experience very quickly. And fortunately Sandi was busy teaching new entrants at a local school. We lived near to the hospital, so I could keep in close contact with Sandi, but still, it was hard on her — being a doctor's wife sounds good in theory, but it certainly has its drawbacks.

Medicine is a constant reminder of the big mysteries of the human condition, but there's nothing like your own pregnancy and childbirth. In 1984 we were both rapt when Sandi had a positive pregnancy test. For quite a while nothing much changed, except Sandi and I spent a lot of our spare time shopping for all the shit that parents need to raise a child in the First World. Much of the rest of our time was spent speculating about the little alien growing inside her. Would it be handsome and intelligent, like Sandi? Would it be tall, rugged and charming? Or would it be like me? Would it be a boy or a girl? Fair- or dark-haired? What colour eyes would it have, and when could I take it hunting?

Soon there was no doubt that this was not an exercise, as Sandi's tummy started growing outwards and upwards. We progressively told our friends, many of whom — mostly being of the chardonnay set (childless and happy that way) — reacted with a mixture of sympathy and horror. Pregnancy and parenthood, as we discovered, are very much you-have-to-have-been-there experiences, like other natural disasters, or war. As for childbirth itself, despite my stint working in obstetrics, I went into the delivery suite imagining my loved one sobbing her way through what looked like a prolonged — often hours-long — orgasm while I patted her hand and mopped her brow. I wasn't at all prepared for the bloody, visceral, traumatic horror show that it really is, and I'm not sure Sandi was either.

Pretty early on, I began to realise why they call it 'labour' rather than something else, like 'holiday' or 'lots of laughs', and to understand why one in 20 women as recently as 100 years ago didn't make it through the business. Never mind Sandi, I was exhausted by the end of it, and hardly had the energy for authentic emotion when they handed me my crimson, bloody, bellowing daughter. But I was conscious of joy, and afterwards — quite soon afterwards, when I was exercising my male prerogative and recovering with a medicinal beer — the joy grew to be quite intense. I was pleased I was a dad, nearly as pleased as I was that my role in the whole procreation business had been that of the male. I might even have said a silent prayer of thanks, and added — while I had the ear of whatever deity was listening — that if it were possible to choose, I'd really rather come back as a male in any prospective future lives, if it was all the same to the management.

If labour was scary, then what came next was positively terrifying. Sandi and I found ourselves blinking in the Hutt Valley sunshine with a real live baby in our care, Niki. It felt like there must have been some sort of mistake. We couldn't possibly be trusted with this job: we didn't have the faintest clue what we were doing. I experienced acute flashbacks to my first day on the orthopaedics ward, wearing my doctor badge on my chest. Who in their right mind would trust me with a 'Dad' badge? Luckily, we had amazing support from day one from Sandi's folks, Don and Jenny, who lived in Whanganui, and Granny Olive, who was living in Paraparaumu at the time.

This was also where the husband-and-wife teamwork came in for us. Every relationship is different and what works for one couple won't work for another. I've been with Sandi for nearly 40 years now, and in all that time, I've never cooked a dinner or done any housework. That might make me sound like a deluxe a-woman's-place-is-in-the-home Neanderthal, but I swear it's not the case. Both of us happily did our own thing, with Sandi making the house a home and me earning the dosh, which meant I worked long hours, either studying or getting to grips with medicine. Sometimes we'd even meet in the hall between jobs.

Once the kids started turning up and life became more of a zoo, our teamwork really saved the day. Sandi did an awesome job, and she spared me many a dose of sleep deprivation and fatigue from being up and down like a yoyo sorting out squealing kids late at night.

＝

Despite working hard at Hutt Hospital and learning to be a first-time dad, I did manage — with Sandi's blessing — to sneak out into the bush for the odd deer-hunting trip to keep my sanity. It must have been around this time that one of my more memorable hunting stories occurred.

It all started when a really cool bloke and a great mate of mine by the name of Dr Malcolm Abernethy suggested we go hunting. We met up after work, with a general plan of driving about an hour north of Wellington to Otaki Forks and heading off up the Waitewaewae Hut track to see what we could find to shoot around the Waitewaewae Flats. Naturally I took along my regular hunting companion, Camellia, but Mal seemed to take an instant dislike to her. In fact, he rather unkindly referred to her as a 'bush rat' and suggested she belonged at home with corgis and other such lapdogs.

After we had walked for an hour or so, I realised I wasn't enjoying myself as much as normal. I usually revelled in the sounds of the New Zealand wilderness: the river chuckling in its stony bed, the wind sighing through the bush and it all punctuated by the beautiful, ringing calls of native birds. But it was cancelled out somehow by Malcolm's constant, low-grade muttering about my gorgeous little hound. Camellia wasn't bothered: after all, dogs are Buddhists by nature, repelling any negative energy with soulful, eternal positivity. She greeted every dark look and cuss word from Mal with vigorous wagging of her curly tail, which just seemed to get even further up Mal's nose.

Luckily for everyone, the walk in to our campsite wasn't too long. We set up just before dark and got a good fire going to make our tea. We discussed our plan of action for the morning's hunting.

'I'm keen to have a crack at a stag,' Mal said. 'Know any good spots around here?'

I thought about it and, as a matter of fact, I did. Some were easy to get to. Some were quite a lot harder. And of course I also had to factor in everything Mal had said about my dog . . .

'Well, probably the best spot would be up the Otaki a bit. There's some flats up there where you see the big boys from time to time. Just head upstream. You come to a little gorge with a bit of a waterfall. The flats are just up past there.'

I'd swear Camellia shot me a wink.

After we'd eaten and washed up, we climbed into our sleeping bags. It was too cold to sit around. Out of habit, I held my bag open for Camellia to burrow down inside and curl up, nice and warm, against me.

At about two in the morning, I was woken by a sharp prod in the side.

'Jeez, it's cold,' bleated Malcolm. 'Can I borrow the dog?'

'I thought you hated the dog,' I mumbled.

'Nah, I love the dog!' he protested.

I did my Christian duty and dug out Camellia and handed her over to Mal. She looked around blearily as her new bed mate gratefully stuffed her into his own bag. Even when she let rip with one of her trademark monster farts, he didn't have a word to say against her.

'Talk about changing your tune, Mal,' I said, but the only reply was a gentle snore.

In the early morning darkness, we got up and got going. Mal headed upriver to the fabled stag ground I had told him of and Camellia and I walked to the rather more mellow terrain of the Waitewaewae Flats. I shot a deer with my Mohawk .222 over 400 metres, a nice young hind that promised good eating.

Camellia and I were already back at camp feeling pretty pleased with ourselves by the time the sun eventually heaved over the Tararua Range and burned off the last of the chilly mist hanging in the river valley. It was some time before Mal showed up, empty-handed, soaked to the skin and shivering violently.

'Little gorge?' he shrieked through chattering teeth. 'Niagara fucken Falls, you mean! You prick!'

I feigned innocence and frowned. 'You must have taken a wrong turn.' Camellia wagged her tail and blinked up at me in that adoring way that dogs do, as if to let me know that my secret was safe with her.

The trouble with finding every single one of my hospital runs so fascinating and engaging was that I reached the end of my two years as a house surgeon in 1985 without any clear notion of what, if anything, I'd like to specialise in. Apart from what golf club to belong to, specialisation is probably the hardest question in any medical career. You invest so much time and effort in your training that it's pretty hard to go back once you've committed yourself to a particular discipline. The mistake that too many young doctors make is to choose too soon and discover they've made a mistake only after they've gone too far down the road and qualified. I didn't want to fall into that trap. Toss in the complicating fact that there are over 50 disciplines and sub-disciplines to which you can devote yourself, and it's not an easy call to make.

Luckily, rather than be a master of any particular trade, you can choose to be jack of all of them, and that's what I thought I'd do. I would be a general practitioner. I hadn't forgotten Dr Jacobsen drifting before a warm, rum-scented breeze in his whaleboat: on the contrary, over the past two years I'd thought of him every time I finished a nightshift, bone-weary and wondering whether it was all worthwhile. Perhaps I, too, could fit general practice around the loves of my life rather than the other way round.

By now I was also aware that I preferred the idea of continuity of care over the kind of production-line patient encounters that the hospital system provides. As a hospital doctor you see a patient only for as long as you need to in order to fix their particular, immediate problem. As a GP you form ongoing, often lifelong relationships with your patients: you are stuck with them, to put it bluntly, and they are stuck with you. I suppose I was finding out that I was a people person; building long-term relationships seemed like an attractive prospect.

There are some personalities in the profession who feel that as soon as you have achieved registration as a medical practitioner (which happens after a year as a house surgeon) you're qualified to hang up one's shingle and go into business as a general practitioner. And in those days, the law happened to agree. But I was not of that opinion: when I thought about what it would be like to open the door to a waiting room full of patients, each with a more or less obscure complaint, I suffered the same self-doubt that I had on day one of being a house surgeon. Although the last thing I wanted to do was more training, I decided it wouldn't be silly to enrol in the training scheme for GPs, the Primex course, established by the relatively young Royal New Zealand College of

General Practitioners. I had an inkling that membership would stand me in good stead later on in my professional life. Most trades and professions tend to become more regulated over time, and I thought it made sense to be part of the in-crowd from the start. I applied for the course and was accepted.

The year-long GP Primex course was conveniently located in Lower Hutt, and was run by a pair of doctors, Dr Pete Anyon and Dr Humphrey Rainey. Along with 14 other aspiring GPs from a wide variety of backgrounds, I enrolled in the class of 1987 and had a good feeling right from the start. Dr Pete and Dr Humphrey were a real hoot, both open-minded and approachable; you could voice any opinion on the course material whatsoever, whether you agreed with them or not, without fear of them getting their backs up. They created a relaxed, collegial atmosphere.

Besides giving us some insight into what it was like to handle a regular patient clientele — none of us, with our hospital training, had a clue about this — the course introduced us to the many and varied approaches to health and well-being out there in the community. We met lots of interesting people, from politicians and physiotherapists to chiropractors and faith healers, and so far as we could tell, Dr Pete and Dr Humphrey were completely open-minded about all of them (even the politicians). One of the most reassuring aspects of the course for me, still agonising over whether I'd made the right decision to go into general practice, was that these two very cool individuals, both with solid hospital specialist experience (in their former lives, Dr Pete was a paediatrician and Dr Humphrey was an anaesthetist), had chosen to become GPs instead. So the job must have something going for it!

By now, though, I had seriously itchy feet. I was ready for my future to begin. After five years at varsity, two years in the hospital and now midway through another year in GP school, I had the very real sense that all work and no play was making me a very dull boy. The effort of setting hopes and dreams aside and keeping my mind on the job had taken its toll, and I was ready to start planning my future again. I think all of us on the course felt the same and, as the year progressed, we were conscious of a growing sense that the Promised Land was at hand.

Conversations were dominated by discussion and debate about the relative merits of the different kinds of practice we thought we'd have once we were unleashed upon the real world; I enjoyed listening to the various dreams and schemes that people had — setting up shop in rural areas or in posh consulting rooms in 'the big smoke', perhaps even central Wellington. But nothing I heard made me waver at all from The Jacobsen Plan. All I wanted was to be my own boss like Dr Jacobsen, messing about in boats down there in the Sounds, with enough freedom to pursue his passions and interests. And so much the better, in my case, if those interests had a decent sets of antlers.

During my time training as a GP, Sandi and I seemed to have a bit more social time on our hands. That meant lots more gatherings with our mates were on the cards and the start of lifelong friendships with my fellow trainees. Life was pretty good.

Unfortunately, during these years of hard yakka, my poor old dad was going downhill. Most of us harbour regrets about not spending enough time with family members on the slippery slope, and I wish I had sat down with Dad more often. Despite starting to lose his short-term memory and getting a bit dithery, he never lost his sense of humour and was fun to be with to the end. He still had so many good stories to tell, and some of them were probably true.

His demise was mercifully quick when it came. He had a fall and fractured his hip, and while in hospital he developed pneumonia and died painlessly. As time has gone on, I have come to realise that I carry many of his traits. That makes me proud.

In April 1987, about halfway through the GP course and during the roar, as it happens, I had the opportunity to test-drive my dream. As trainees on the Primex course, we were encouraged to get practical experience by doing a month of supervised work at a real, live general practice. I made enquiries at the Fiordland Medical Practice at Te Anau, only the gateway to the deer-infested Fiordland National Park and UNESCO-listed World Heritage Area Te Wahipounamu! I chose this place because it had everything I wanted in life: mountains, lakes, bush and every flavour of deer. The place was run by Dr Trevor Walker and Dr Patrick O'Sullivan. They had no hesitation in agreeing to supervise me for a month, and they turned out to be great blokes. I learned a lot from them.

It all got off to a really good start. Pete Devane, a mate from my Forest Service days in the Tararua District, and I stuck our hands up and got allotted the upper Glaisnock River valley roar block 54, and so we got a hunt in before my general practice work actually began. We took a floatplane to North Fiord, one of three arms off the western flank of Lake Te Anau, to get access to the Glaisnock River. We had the pilot buzz us up the valley a bit before we landed on the lake so that we could check out potential campsites. We unloaded our packs and rifles and set off up the river valley to the confluence of Kakapo Creek and the Glaisnock, where we planned to base ourselves. We intended to hunt around the Edith Saddle at the Glaisnock's headwaters.

It was beautiful country. The Glaisnock winds its way, clear and green, along the floor of a broad glacial valley, with steep, bush-clad bluffs rearing on either side and occasional glimpses of snow-capped peaks at its head. Over the next couple of days we hunted in the vicinity of the Kakapo and Takahe streams, but saw no deer, little sign and didn't hear a solitary bugle. It didn't look as though the fabled Glaisnock would live up to its reputation.

By the time we reached the head of the valley, it turned into pretty hard going where we were pushing our way through chest-deep crown fern that was not quite high enough to duck beneath. As we couldn't proceed doubled over with a heavy pack, we couldn't see where the hell we were putting our feet. Given how heavy our packs were, the slightest misstep would send us tits-up into the scrub — and it did, over and over, pitching us into the damp, mossy darkness beneath the ferns. It's only funny the first few hundred times.

I'd already had a gutsful of falling over when I did it again. As I lifted my face from the dirt to curse, my eyes fell upon a strange shape in the gloomy recess under an ancient, fallen tree. I reached out and touched plastic. It was a large, bulging bag. I did the decent thing, pulled it out and investigated, and was rewarded with no fewer than eight canned Colman's Self-Saucing Golden

Syrup Spongy Puds. Pete was impressed. We whooped and did a little dance of joy. Our moral duty was clear, and we wasted no time in stuffing them into our already overloaded packs. We pressed on and, with the help of a solitary hunter we encountered in the scrub, we eventually made the saddle and located the famous rock bivouac where we set up for the next day's hunting. The valley forks here, and we chose a valley each to reconnoitre: I took the lucky left, while Pete headed off to the right. I found a nice slip that led from the valley floor to the mountaintop that was lined by the kinds of juicy grasses that deer love to munch. I was encouraged by a scattering of hefty deer sign. It was looking good for the morning!

Pete had found nothing but bluffs.

At nightfall, when the sandflies finally buggered off, we celebrated with a spongy pud, both of us privately reflecting, I am sure, on the notion of divine providence.

Early in the morning, before Pete was even awake, I snuck off to the slip I had explored the day before. I came over the top of a small, rocky knoll that hid the slope from view and found myself looking at the pale rump of a large wapiti bull from 30 metres' range. I couldn't believe my luck! I slid the bolt of my trusty .243 home and centred the animal in the cross hairs. It was so close I could see the fleas nodding to each other. The obliging wapiti even turned side-on for me; as I waited, it took a further half-step forward, exposing its heart and lung area.

I fired, and it jumped about 10 feet in the air and took off.

What the fuck? What would Pete say when I told him I had missed at point-blank range?

I headed over to where the animal had disappeared into the

bush on the other side of the slip and listened for the tell-tale sounds of a wounded deer crashing its way through the trees.

Nothing.

My mood had gone from elation to complete despair, but when I happened to glance to one side, I saw the deer, dead, just below me.

The rain, which had been threatening for a day or two, now came down in sheets. I hurried back to camp and woke Pete with my wild story and asked him to help. He looked out into the streaming dawn and, true to form, tugged on his clothes and boots and tagged along. I admired his dissection work as he jointed the deer, and we both cooed over the animal's antlers, which had 10 nicely symmetrical points and spanned, I reckoned, a whole metre.

You'd swear Pete had shot it himself, he was so chuffed for me. It was such a buzz, and every deerstalker's dream — collecting a nice head in the middle of the most glorious mountains you could ever imagine.

The rain kept us pinned down in the bivvy for the rest of the day, but as we leisurely dined on fresh venison, sipped Baileys Irish Cream and polished off the remaining spongy puds, Pete and I agreed that things could definitely have been worse.

Once the storm let up, we descended from the Edith Saddle to the valley below and rocked up to the Glaisnock Hut for our final night. We found ourselves sharing it with a party of four stringy, unshaven hunters. Compared with the usual camaraderie of backcountry huts, this lot eyed us darkly, especially when they heard where we had come from.

'You jokers wouldn't happen to have seen a bag of spongy puds hidden in the scrub up there, would you?' one of them asked.

Pete and I assumed expressions of pure, wide-eyed innocence.

'Naaaaah, not us,' I said, spreading my hands wide.

I was only at the Fiordland Medical Practice for a short time, but it was long enough to get a good feel for the place and gain some other insights as a bonus. Amongst the centre's clientele were quite a few of the fabled chopper boys — the bush helicopter pilots I had idolised from my earliest days as a hunter, when I would be slogging through the cold, wet bush out the back of beyond and suddenly, with the characteristic whine of its turbine engine, a Hughes 500D would sweep over me at treetop level, making me instinctively duck to avoid a haircut. It would be a venison crew, pilot and shooter, hard at work in their office.

Cor, I used to think, bet those guys pull the chicks.

I used to imagine living that lifestyle, swooping and soaring like a bird over the more majestic reaches of the New Zealand landscape in search of deer to shoot, returning home rugged and windswept in the evening to the worshipful gazes of my perfect children, the warm embrace of my perfect wife . . . To put it bluntly, I thought the sun shone from the arses of the people who had the balls to live like that.

The reality, as I soon found in their medical files, was quite the opposite. There was one pilot in particular who was on the practice's books: a legend of the venison recovery trade who had been a hero to me in my youth, the way movie stars or rock gods were to others. I read aghast in his notes about the alcoholism, the risk-taking and the long list of broken marriages, failed relationships and depressive episodes that went with them. So much for that hero, then. The gloss was gone for good. Perhaps I was just growing up.

Around this time, I was rostered on one evening as the emergency duty doctor for the region. Early on I got a call from the Queenstown Police saying a tramper had suffered an emergency up on the Routeburn Track and, as it was in my patch, could I shoot up there and sort things out. They thought he might be dead. One of the practice nurses and I immediately drove to the airstrip where a chopper was waiting for us, and it buzzed us off up into the hills. The pilot set us down near a little tarn on a ridge beneath the frowning Humboldt Mountains. We grabbed our emergency gear and scuttled up the track for 10 minutes to the point where the tramper was lying, surrounded by a few members of his family and a worried-looking warden from the hut a kilometre further on.

As I examined the patient — he was a slightly built man in his seventies, cool to the touch, and had no vital signs at all — they told me that he was a university professor who had lately retired. This trip to walk the Routeburn was his retirement present to himself. He had been slow on this section of the track, and had finally told his companions that he was a bit puffed and that they should go on ahead of him. He reckoned he would sit down and smoke a pipe and catch them up at the hut. They did as he asked. The professor had walked a short distance off the track, sat down, loaded his pipe and lit up, then keeled over. When he failed to arrive at the hut, his family had gone looking and found him, his pipe still clutched in his hand, where he had toppled gently off his perch into the tussock.

We couldn't carry him down to the chopper without a stretcher, so the nurse and the hut warden volunteered to go back for it. The dead man's family took their tearful leave of the deceased and walked back off towards the hut, leaving me alone with him for quarter of an hour. I sat beside him and looked around appreciatively. It was a section of the track where the pale green foliage of the ribbonwood trees makes it look like a stonefruit orchard, hence its name, The Orchard. On the margins of the valley, the ribbonwoods give over to beech that climb the steep walls; that day the sky was colouring up behind the mighty, snow-capped Darrans, which presided over the whole scene from the opposite side of the Hollyford Valley.

It occurred to me that none of the professor's family or friends had been too upset, and I could see why. He had lived a long, successful and fulfilling life, and his last moments had been spent at peace in one of the most beautiful places on earth, knowing his family were nearby, safe and happy and perfectly untroubled by his onrushing end. No mouldering away in a rest home for him, and none of the grisly interventions of end-of-life medical care.

'That's the way, mate,' I told him softly, and I knew it was true. That's the way I want to go, too.

… CHAPTER 4 …

HORSEPITAL HERE WE COME

I arrived back from my month's placement at Fiordland Medical Practice champing at the bit. I wanted to finish my GP training and get the exams out of the way so that I could shift my little family to Te Anau and get after those deer again. It was pretty much everything I'd dreamed of: a congenial workplace (which had expressed itself willing to have me), friendly locals and the world's greatest playground right there on my doorstep. It was The Jacobsen Plan just as I'd imagined it, and it was there for the taking.

But talking it over with Sandi brought me back to earth (she's good like that: in any successful relationship, one of you has to be). She was keen to come and be part of the big adventure, but we had to consider the downside, too: it was a big step for someone as young and good-looking as me to lock myself into general practice, especially in such an isolated spot, so far from our ageing parents and all of the opportunities and support that family and large population centres afforded young parents. Sandi was pregnant with Marc, and we both agreed that family support, if you're lucky enough to have it, was too important. With a heavy heart, I dropped the boys in Te Anau a line to let them know they needn't keep my place warm — or at least, not for now.

Exam time came and went at the end of 1987 and I had no problem passing my GP examinations. Now that we had flagged the idea of Te Anau, it occurred to me that if the time was not right to commit to general practice, there would be no harm in having a look at a speciality. I had been told by those in the know that the longer in the tooth you were before you started training, the harder the specialities were. So it seemed like as good a time as any to have a go — after all, you never know till you try, right? On the plus side, there were plenty of specialist trainee positions going at Palmerston North (Te Papaioea) Hospital, which would keep us close to Granny Olive and Sandi's folks in Whanganui. Even if I emerged on the other side of it all firmly convinced it wasn't for me, I knew the extra experience and expertise would never go astray in general practice. It was kind of a win-win from a professional point of view.

My soul squirmed, though, at the thought of more time — years of it, in fact — back in the hospital system with a lot of regular and bloody hard exams, too, by all accounts. My bottom lip must have wobbled, because Sandi definitely looked sorry for me.

'What can you do outside work that will help make you feel better?' she asked.

I didn't have to think about it for very long.

'Fly,' I said promptly. 'I reckon I might try to knock off my private pilot's licence, if I can.'

We Baldwins had grown up with Stan's hairy-chested stories of flying, and the odd little anecdote about crashes and horrific, fiery deaths had done nothing to dampen our dreams. Richard was the first of us to get his private pilot's licence (PPL) in 1977 while he was working as a fireman, and he owned his own plane, a lovingly restored Auster J5B. I hid my jealousy well, but the time seemed right to go for my own wings.

'OK,' said Sandi. 'Good idea.'

So that was the plan. I would have a look at specialising, while I wasn't flying and — I added, in my best negotiator's voice — skipping off for the odd spot of hunting from time to time.

'And who knows?' I added. 'The kids may well want to come along with me as time goes on.'

=

At the end of 1987, a very pregnant Sandi and I loaded up the last of our gear on the wagon, tied Niki to her car seat and stowed the cardboard box containing the cat as far back as we could in the car so we didn't have to listen to her deranged growling and hissing for the whole of our journey. We waved to the small group of friends who had lined up to flutter handkerchiefs as we pulled out of our street.

The most common response to our announcement that we were upping sticks and leaving the Hutt Valley to return to Palmerston North was a stunned 'Why?' Some people tried to talk us out of it. A few wept openly, as though we had told them we were off on a desperate journey with only a slim chance of survival. I must admit, I had a lump in my throat as I looked back at 99 Witako Street in the rear-view mirror. Our first child had been born there. We had achieved so much there. Perhaps we were, as our friends suggested, mad to be leaving. Or perhaps we were simply mad to be going to Palmerston North. Some of them had suggested that, too.

Despite this, Sandi and I were both excited about this new chapter in our adventure, and we had no trouble settling back into Palmy. Sandi had already found us a home, a little cottage close to Russell Street School (which had a very good reputation) and a hop, skip and a jump from Palmerston North Hospital, or 'Horsepital' as it was universally known in the Baldwin family, commemorating my struggles with spelling as a wayward and possibly dyslexic child. With the hospital handy I could easily shoot home while I was doing the after-hours on-call roster. In fact, the only member of the family who seemed to find the new arrangement suboptimal was the cat, who went from being master of her own Lower Hutt domain to just another contender in the feline gangland that was Langston Avenue and its environs.

A couple of days after we had shifted in, I strolled up the steps of the big old main building of the horsepital, shrugged into a white coat and pinned on my shiny new name badge, which read: 'Dr D. Baldwin — General Medical Registrar'. The genius of the medical education system is that at every step of the way, they dangle the carrot of qualifications in front of you while making you work the hospital treadmill, doing all the donkey doctor work that is beneath the dignity of the specialists. It would take the best part of two years as a general medical registrar before I could sit the exams that would steer me into a speciality. At that point, I had a wide choice: neurology (brains and nerves), gastroenterology (guts), nephrology (kidneys), rheumatology (joints and arthritis) or cardiology (hearts and blood vessels), to name but a few. By the time those two years were over, the health system would have had its pound of flesh out of me; I would have to deal with whatever walked through the door and, generally speaking, that meant anyone who was too sick or complicated to be dealt with in the primary health sector (that is, by GPs out there in the community). It promised to be very valuable experience, whatever happened down the track.

Still, I wasn't exactly thrilled to be back in an institution. Because I had indicated a vague interest in specialising in it, I was assigned to cardiology. My first impression of my new boss wasn't favourable: he was nattily dressed, complete with a bow tie. My second impression wasn't much better: he spoke with a posh Pommy accent and we'd hardly been talking five minutes before he dropped a few dozen names to show he was well in with the great and the good. He was what dear old Stan would have called a toff, and frankly, I couldn't see us getting along. Still, his first impressions of me were hardly likely to have been any more favourable. My first words to him were: 'Where can I get a bloody coffee around this dump?' He looked highly defensive of the cafeteria ladies. Our first day was marked with verbal clashes of one sort or another. I'm sure both he and I went home thinking that it was looking like it might be a very long five years — the time it takes to specialise.

Our relationship began to thaw one night when I got the call to go to accident and emergency, where an ambulance was due to bring in a patient in full cardiac arrest. The ambulance was already pulling in when I arrived, and I yanked open the doors to find two huge paramedics working frantically on the patient, huffing and puffing like steam engines. I jumped up and down, craned my neck, ducked and weaved, but no matter what I tried, I couldn't so much as get a glimpse of the patient past the heaving, sweating paramedics. Then one of them planted his feet a little further apart to get better purchase on the chest compressions he was administering and, without thinking twice, I dived between his massive thighs. When my head popped out from his crutch he did a double take then jumped so high he hit his head on the roof, clamping his legs together as he did. Shaking his head against the pain, he planted his palm on the crown of my head and pushed me backwards. I popped out and landed 'splat' on the tarmac behind the ambulance like a white-coated turd.

Three was clearly a crowd in the ambulance.

'Let's get him out of there!' I yelled, and they bundled the patient out of the ambulance and positioned him on the A&E resuscitation bed and began wheeling it into the Emergency Room. The usual crowd of paramedics, orderlies and the nurses and doctors of the crash team, experts in emergency resuscitation, gathered. As the patient was intubated, intravenous lines inserted and heart-monitoring electrodes taped to his chest, I asked the paramedics for a bit of history.

'Middle-aged male. Attempted suicide,' they said. 'Tried to

gas himself in his car. The engine was still running and he was unresponsive when we reached him.'

By now, the heart monitor was up and running and showing the flattest of flatlines. The crash team were busily administering adrenalin and warming up the defibrillator paddles when my Pommy boss showed up. I stepped out of the ruck, took him next door and gave him a quick rundown.

'He's not responding,' I said. 'I don't get it, because his colour's good, he looks to be in reasonable shape and there are no scars or obvious indications of underlying disease.'

He nodded curtly, went through and elbowed his way into the scrum. He spent a couple of seconds examining the patient. He was back beside me almost immediately.

'What do you think?' I asked, surprised he had been so quick.

He shook his head. 'I think we should call it a day.'

'Why?'

He fixed me in his stare, a slightly amused twinkle in his eye.

'Because he has rigor mortis, you twit,' he whispered, with a slight grin.

I suddenly registered that the patient's limbs had been quite stiff when I performed my initial examination. Rigor mortis sets in between three and four hours after death. And only now did I remember that one of the classic signs of carbon monoxide poisoning was the healthy pink flush it produces on the skin.

Oh shit, I thought. Damn.

My boss was strutting up the corridor; I wouldn't have been surprised if he'd done a little skip and clicked his heels. But I was very conscious of the opportunity he had just — very generously — given me, and I seized it with both hands.

Squaring my shoulders, I strode masterfully into the resuscitation room and ordered everyone to stop work. This was greeted with howls of disapproval and protest.

'Look at his colour—'

'One more shot of adrenalin will do it—'

'Are you mad?'

But I moved forward, turning off the heart monitor with one hand and lifting the dead man's stiff left arm with the other, before proclaiming loudly: 'He has rigor mortis, everyone. He must have been dead for hours.'

There was a brief silence. As I slung my stethoscope over my shoulder, spun on my heel and strode briskly from the room, the whispering started.

'Of course!'

'Why didn't we spot that?'

'So young, but so talented . . .'

'Genius . . .'

'Thanks, boss,' I muttered to myself.

After our rough start, I came to respect and then really like the man. He had an excellent dry wit, which he frequently used to defuse tense situations. And you had to admire his attitude to work. He was no shirker: no matter what day or time it was, and whether he was on or off duty, if he was needed, he was there.

Besides the satisfying variety of work that horsepital offered, it was an excellent work environment to be in, too, in those days.

HORSEPITAL HERE WE COME

One of Palmerston North's greatest assets was the camaraderie that existed amongst all of the doctors working at the hospital, from the lowest house surgeon to the most senior consultants. Everyone was very supportive of one other, and we enjoyed each other's company.

At ten o'clock each morning, everyone who could would meet up for morning tea in the large combined medical staff/smoko room. I really looked forward to these occasions, as the room was always packed with doctors scoffing scones and spilling coffee all over themselves as they waved their hands about and argued about everything from politics to gardening with great vigour. It was noisy and fun.

At that time, home was hardly any quieter. Our second child, Marc, was born on 29 December 1987, and a couple of years later we added Anna to the list of dependants. All of a sudden, we were a family of five with three under-five-year-olds. Our little house wasn't as full with people as the smoko room at work, but you'd be forgiven for thinking it was if you went by the noise.

Parenting young children is like war: you have to have lived through it to understand the levels of noise and terror. At any one point in space and time, a sample of house noise could be taken and it would include a combination of laughter, crying, yelling, giggles, sniffing, screaming, chatter, TV, music, barking dogs and meowing cats, all vying for the honour of being the loudest. I had a whole new respect for Granny Olive, who at one point had coped with four kids pretty much single-handed. Just about all that keeps you going at times is schadenfreude, which I'm pretty sure is the German term for the sadistic thrill you get when you reflect that other young parents of your acquaintance have it just as bad, or worse. Special bonds are forged on the front lines of raising infants: the dark rings under the eyes, the greying hair, the streak of sick on the shoulder, the faint whiff of very second-hand nappies . . . They mark you out to others as comrades in the whole harrowing and joyous business, as surely as an RSA badge identifies one veteran to another, inspiring nods of mutual recognition. We too served and we know. The bonds of friendship formed during this time of your life are deeper than the shallow acquaintances you make on the sports field, or in the classroom, or staggering around the sticky carpet at the Fitz. Many of the people who helped us at that stage of our lives, and whom we helped in turn, are still our dearest friends to this day.

The true survivor — the only member of the family who positively thrived though this period — was Camellia. She would appear whenever we signalled dinner time by laying tarpaulins over the carpet. All three of ours were relatively good eaters (assuming some proportion of what was smeared on their faces at mealtimes actually made it into their mouths) but none of them were quick to catch on to the finer points of table manners, and they seemed to have silently agreed amongst themselves that the best way to signal to us that they had had enough was to use their food, drink or utensils as projectiles.

Camellia would lurk beneath the table, or under one or other of the highchairs, ready to pounce on whatever manna rained from heaven, but she had to be careful: like all blessings in this vale of tears, these were mixed and could come with the occasional knife, fork, plate or cup. She suffered a few nasty blows early on in the piece, but proved herself resilient and highly adaptable; she soon learned how to move unerringly to anything edible while keeping a weather eye out for hard objects. The symbiotic relationship she developed with our kids at feeding time reminded me of those crafty little birds you see on the Discovery Channel that hop around inside the mouths of crocodiles, picking food from between sharp teeth and somehow knowing exactly when to hop out before the croc snaps its jaws shut.

Despite a very busy work and family life, I still managed to find the time to get out to the airfield for flying lessons. My first flight was with Chester Rowles in a United Aviation-owned Piper PA-38 Tomahawk registered ZK-KVM on 17 January 1988. In perfect weather we zoomed about Manawatu's airspace learning 'the effect of controls'. I was hooked. It was the absolute opposite of being stuck in a classroom, or at the horsepital. It was everything I had dreamed it would be when my soul soared with the seagulls outside the windows of Paremata School.

We coasted over the foothills of the Tararuas, covering in seconds what it had taken me hours to slog over on foot on my early hunting expeditions, and I sensed the possibilities that my pilot's licence would offer up. I found time to show up for lessons most days with Chester or Rod Buchanan and Bob Swanney, the other two instructors at United Aviation. I loved every minute of the compulsory 50 hours' flight time I had to acquire in order to sit my licence.

My first solo was pretty cool, but nothing compared with the moment when Bob Swanney told me I could take the Piper out on SORJ — standard overhead rejoin — which meant that I could leave the boring old circuit we had flown again and again for the first time. On SORJ, you're meant to fly about five nautical miles from the airport and then return to join the circuit in the correct pattern. But, hell, it was my first taste of real freedom! I had been too busy holding onto the aircraft to really enjoy my first solo, but this time I was ecstatic. The five miles might have easily stretched out to become 15, and I had to fight the urge to keep going, to head off into the hills and do some exploring.

I sat and passed my PPL on 1 June 1988 with a very experienced examiner, Peter Kidd, in the hot seat at Hastings Airport. Peter looked pretty dubious about the standard of maintenance of the United Aviation aircraft I turned up in, and I thought I might have stuffed up when I got a bit over-vigorous with my wing-drop stall recovery and Peter banged his head hard on the cockpit roof. But headache notwithstanding (and no pun intended) Peter passed me with flying colours.

Pretty much as soon as I landed back at Palmy, I got Rob Buchanan to check me out for my Cessna 172 rating — a 'type rating' is the extra hoop a qualified pilot has to jump through to show they know how to handle a particular aircraft. I had initially learnt to fly in a Piper Tomahawk, so I had to get checked out for the Cessna. The idea was that I could use the four-seater 172 to take family and friends on sightseeing rides or even little trips away from Palmy, such as over to Blenheim where all those lovely vineyards are. It was the beginning of a love affair with Cessna aircraft that continues to this day.

HORSEPITAL HERE WE COME

I don't know how committed I was to qualifying as a cardiologist. I was interested in cardiology because I had always been interested in the heart. As a kid, I occasionally noticed that even after some of the animals I had caught — ducks, fish or rabbits — had been killed and gutted, there would still be some activity in the heart. I was fascinated by those weird little throbbing things, and tried various methods of keeping them going a bit longer, but none of them (not even pouring warm water on them or poking them with a stick) seemed to do the trick.

Granny Olive was partial to venison hearts, and she would sometimes cook sheep hearts for breakfast. I would volunteer to cut them up so that I could look inside them and have a bit of a fiddle around. The intricate papillary muscle and valve anatomy never ceased to amaze me. Plus they tasted so bloody good, too.

I renewed my fascination with this amazing organ in the physiology papers I did for my science degree. So now, when forced to work out which bit of the body I would specialise in treating as a doctor, the heart seemed like the natural choice.

But perhaps the heart I came to know best was my own, when I worked out that it wasn't really into specialising, after all. It's not often we're presented with the choices that we have to make in life in quite such clearly defined terms, but as it turned out, my physician exams that I needed to pass in order to become a cardiologist were scheduled to clash directly with my PPL exams. I didn't have to think too long or hard: I sat my PPL. The die, in many ways, was cast.

One fine Saturday morning, when I had just arrived at work, the emergency department called me to attend to a patient who'd just wandered in with symptoms suggestive of a heart attack. I duly rushed down the stairs and straight into the Emergency Room, where I found a middle-aged Maori male. He had clearly been quite a physical specimen, with the build of a warrior gone to seed. He was covered in scars and tattoos, right down to the obligatory LOVE and HATE inked on his knuckles. The tats really stood out, as he was paler than the average honky due to poor blood flow to his skin. The fierce impression his appearance made was softened, though, by the big smile he gave me, despite being in obvious pain.

'Gidday, doc,' he said, in a soft, friendly voice.

He — let's call him Tama — told me he had first started having chest pain during the night, but he hadn't wanted to bother anyone. I took his history and all the indications were bleak: he was a smoker, he was overweight and pretty much every male member of his extended family had died under the age of 60 from heart attacks or heart failure due to rheumatic fever.

I examined Tama and ran an electrocardiogram that, sure enough, showed he'd suffered a significant anterior heart attack. While I was reviewing his results, he lost consciousness and his heart went into what we brainy bastards call ventricular fibrillation, meaning the muscles of the lower chambers start to quiver spasmodically instead of performing the strong, steady throb (the sinus rhythm) that they do when they're working properly. This is usually fatal. But Tama had chosen a good spot for it: he was lying in an A&E centre on a resuscitation bed with lots of highly trained staff at hand, two working intravenous lines in place for the administration of life-saving drugs and, oh yes, a cardiac defibrillator right beside him. I grabbed the defibrillator paddles, applied them to his chest, turned the volume right up and gave him both barrels — a 360-joule shock. He jerked stiff with the electric shock, but soon relaxed; his heart settled back into its normal sinus rhythm and his circulation returned.

A minute or so later, Tama came around. His hand went searchingly to his chest. 'Shit, bro,' he said. 'What was that all about?'

'You were on your way to meet Jesus,' I told him, because although I'd only known him for 15 minutes, some of which he'd spent dead, I knew we were going to hit it off.

'Not so sure I'll be going that way,' he chuckled. 'Few skeletons in the closet!'

'Join the club, Tama,' I said, as the house surgeon gave him a cocktail of drugs to relieve the pain and prevent another arrhythmia. We also wanted to sedate him for a while. He slipped into sleep while we shifted him upstairs to the coronary care unit (CCU).

As the morning wore on, Tama went into cardiac arrest four more times in the CCU. Each time, I dropped whatever I was doing and rushed from wherever I was to help resuscitate him. He responded to the cardiac defibrillation each time, but it was obvious this wasn't going to go on forever. His heart muscle was damaged and was electrically unstable. It was very likely to tip over into fatal heart arrhythmia at any moment, and even the drugs we had to control that kind of carry-on were far from fail-safe.

Each time Tama woke after being resuscitated he was quite

chirpy. He didn't seem fazed at all, even when I explained to him what was going on and how serious his condition was.

'Do you want me to contact anyone?' I asked. 'Family, whoever?'

'Nah,' he said cheerfully. 'I don't want to put anyone to any bother.'

I rang my Pommy cardiologist boss for advice on how to handle the situation, and to ask if there were any other drugs he could think of that might help stabilise Tama's heart.

'From those results,' he said, 'the poor sod's heart's buggered. There comes a point where medicine has to give way to miracles if you're going to keep someone alive. You can keep zapping him if you like, but it's not going to change the outcome. Your call on that one. Sorry,' he added.

I told the rest of the CCU staff the grim news and to hold off on any further resuscitation attempts until I had talked to Tama. By now, I'd had the pleasure of knowing him for six hours, but we were getting on as though we'd been mates all our lives. He had a huge repertoire of funny stories and a real talent for delivering them. We spent much of the time I was supposed to be talking about medical matters talking about everything but, both of us in stitches.

His face lit up when I drew back the curtain to his cubicle, and I forced a smile in return. I sat down and gave him the bad news.

'Sorry, mate, but you've had a series of pretty bad heart attacks. The muscle of your heart is damaged, which is why it keeps conking out. We can jump-start it and get it going again, but it's not going to work in the long term. How long do you want us to keep doing it? I'll keep going all night if I have to, but it's your call, in the end.'

He looked perfectly serene. 'Don't worry about it, bro,' he said casually. 'Let's just call it a day there.'

'Are you sure?' I said, and he nodded.

'Yeah. Just means I'll catch up with my mates in the sky. Plenty of them up there.'

I was humbled by his attitude. So often, you see people fighting to keep whatever it is they value — family, in most cases, but sometimes inconsequential stuff like material possessions or status and big-shot reputations. Not for Tama. We talked about it, and as we did, I noticed the heart monitor showing a sudden change from the normal sinus rhythm to ventricular fibrillation. I didn't say anything to Tama, who was talking as though nothing was happening. After 15 seconds or so, he started to slow down and slur his words as the blood flow to his brain slowed. Tama blinked slowly, stopped talking, and then his eyes focused on me in a strong, direct stare.

'See you round, bro,' he said simply, and with that his eyes closed and his head slowly relaxed, turning to the left. He was dead. I performed the usual checks, turned off the heart monitor and then moved off to a side room where for ages I could do nothing but bawl my eyes out. I had only known him for a very short time, and yet I was conscious of a big hole in my life. He was a kindred spirit, no matter how different our lives, backgrounds and experiences had been. And whatever skeletons he had in the closet, I know a good bastard when I see one, and the world always mourns one of those — let alone a human being who can face their death with such courage.

Haere ra, Tama. See you in the next life, buddy.

CHAPTER 5

THE SOLDIER IN ME

Although the work at the horsepital was a great experience, the thought of having to spend the rest of my working life in one big building was starting to turn a bit nightmarish. Making it worse was seeing the mountains and the independence I yearned for directly through most windows. Strictly in accordance with the Law of Greener Pastures, I began to regret my time out from general practice.

As I gazed out at the mountains and thought about my future, I was often distracted by the sound of jet engines thundering overhead. RNZAF Base Ohakea, where New Zealand's strike aircraft were stationed, was just down the road, and eventually it occurred to me that I could join Her Majesty's Gentleman Fighters Club (as the air force had always rather snobbishly distinguished itself from the not-so-gentlemanly navy and the decidedly rough-as-guts army). Dad's reminiscences about life on base were in my thoughts: his occasional observations about how cushy life as base medical officer appeared to be were also front of mind. If nothing else, it promised to offer a completely different experience of medicine, and so I started to make enquiries.

It turned out that the air force was desperate for a base medical officer at RNZAF Base Ohakea, as the incumbent was about to leave. When I expressed interest they were as keen as mustard to get me on board. That level of desperation should have made me suspicious; it seemed the only hurdle was my having to do a four-month Initial Officer Training Course, which was held at RNZAF Base Wigram down in Christchurch. I got in touch with a couple of doctors I knew — Dave Powell and John Welsh — who had previously done the training course, and they talked me through it. It didn't sound as though it would be a barrel of laughs, but it didn't sound impossible either. A lot of soul-searching and chewing it over with Sandi ensued. If she was puzzled or impatient at my apparent inability to settle into anything for an extended period of time, she never showed it. We both sort of knew medical specialisation wasn't for me, and the fall-back position was that if I got court-martialled at officer school or if being a base medical officer simply didn't work out for me, I could always revert to The Jacobsen Plan and buy into a rural GP practice somewhere. And if she was daunted at the prospect of being left alone with the three monsters for nearly five months, she didn't show that, either.

So with Sandi's support, I tendered my resignation at Palmerston North and signed up for RNZAF IOTC 889 (Initial

Officer Training Course August 1989). I thought I had made a bold decision. The opinion of my mates and colleagues was that their suspicions were true: I *was* mad, after all. They had made enquiries about having me committed to a mental institution, they told me, but fortunately my reputation had preceded me and no self-respecting mental health facility would have me. After a while, they went all quiet, and I thought they had accepted my decision and would let me leave unmolested.

Yeah, as they say, right.

=

On my last evening at horsepital, I was walking down the main corridor when a suspiciously large and organised-looking group of junior medical staff and burly orderlies appeared. I realised too late the trouble I was in. They jumped me, and although I put up a valiant struggle, they had soon stripped me and buckled me into an old-fashioned straitjacket. That took care of my torso. An outsized pot of K-Y Jelly, plainly purloined from an ultrasound suite, was produced along with a sack of feathers whose origins were obscure, and I was soon liberally coated from toe to tummy button with both. Then, with no regard for my innocence nor my self-respect, they paraded me through the wards in a distressed and semi-naked state as if I were a criminal heading for the guillotine. The patients thought it was all a great laugh and some got into the spirit and poked me with their walking sticks.

It began to dawn on me as we neared the radiology wing that I was destined for a barium enema (where a mildly radioactive substance is hosed into your colon via the rectum to assist X-ray imaging of potential blockages). I struggled as hard as I could but the straps around me were too tight. Just before we reached the radiology department with its big rubber tube all lubed up and ready to go, I was laid out on the A&E floor for one more ribbing from the staff. As some of my mates — ex-mates now, I vowed — held me down, an orderly climbed over me to retighten a strap. With one last, desperate effort, I worked a hand free of my bonds and grabbed his nuts. He screeched and would have hit the roof, except that his nuts weren't overly large so I had him pretty firmly anchored. There was a sort of stand-off, with everyone telling everyone else to let go. The orderly was now very much on my side, and soon enough I was released from the straitjacket. I slowly released my iron grip on his scrotum and he gingerly slunk off to recover while I got up, all covered in slime and feathers, to give as many people a cuddle as I could. Everyone scattered, but I hunted them down and made them pay.

Sheesh! So much for fond farewells and goodbye presents. I'd have settled for a gold watch.

On 20 August 1989 I waved goodbye to my teary-eyed family at Palmerston North Airport and boarded an Air Nelson Saab bound for Christchurch. It was a short flight, with magnificent views of the snow-covered Alps for much of the way. I was too busy feeling excited and terrified to enjoy the vista as much as I usually would.

Once on the ground I jumped in a taxi for the 15-minute ride to RNZAF Base Wigram, where I presented myself and was directed to join my 10 fellow cadets. I was older than all of them. Those who were closer to my own age were senior non-commissioned officers (NCOs) who were already employed by the RNZAF and who were seen as good officer material. The rest, the real babies, were direct-entry air force cadets who were destined to carry on to a variety of trades, such as engineering or the 'wings' course (aircrew training) once they'd passed officer training. It occurred to me that whereas I had enjoyed a little bit of mana as a senior medical registrar — not to mention a more than half-decent salary — it all counted for nothing here. I was back among the bottom feeders, with hardly more status than a boy scout.

Still, as I reminded myself, I had signed up for this, and coming down in the world was simply the price that had to be paid. Sometimes you have to go back to go forward. I clung to that thought as they issued me with my uniform and ordered me to line up and have my head shaved. I watched in the mirror as my glorious blond locks fell away and I was transformed from free-spirited Dr Dave Baldwin, dad of three, into the slightly nervous-looking Officer Cadet D. E. Baldwin W93568.

Once we were delivered, newly shorn, to our initial mustering station, the warrant officer introduced himself, told us what to expect in terms of our new routine and gave us a rundown of the rules on base. Then he set about deciding who would be temporary NCO — boss cadet — for a week. His beady eyes and accusing finger lighted on me, and it was as though the clouds had split and a burning ray of sunshine had illuminated me . . . *me* amongst all others. Power! Mine, all mine, and for a whole week, too.

My first duty was to march the assembled group of cadets to our barracks. I had no idea how to march, but I didn't let that worry me. And while I could have accomplished this first task quickly and efficiently by marching everyone in a straight line to the barracks, I wanted to savour my first taste of command. I zig-zagged my bemused minions this way and that across the parade ground, in and out of the service buildings and around various obstacles as our warrant officer doubtless watched with an exhausted sense of how big a task he faced bringing this lot up to scratch.

When we eventually reached the barracks, we had three hours to make ready for our first inspection, which we knew was going to be carried out by a grumpy female sergeant. While my authority had been conferred on me by something like divine right, the true leader amongst us — every group has one — soon emerged. One of our fellow cadets, who had invited us all to call him Bucko, stepped up to direct operations. Once we had taken care of our personal responsibilities — neatly stowing our clothes and personal effects and making our beds according to exacting military standards — Bucko had the idea that we should divvy up the rest of the duties instead of tackling each task as a group. This was fine in theory, but Bucko somehow designated me IOTC 889's Chief Ironer of Uniforms. I tried to protest that I didn't have the necessary training for this complex task, but it fell on deaf ears. They showed me the ironing board and iron, pointed at the pile of shirts and trousers and left me to it.

I'd never used a clothes iron in my life. It took me an hour to work out how to turn the fucking thing on, and once I had, it was plain it was going to take a whole lot longer for me to grasp even the bare basics of ironing. Time was running out. I only managed to pass the thing over a few shirts, which looked very much the worse for it, while it hissed and spat derisively. All too soon, everyone came running in to retrieve their uniforms to put them on.

There was a shocked silence. Bucko's shirt was one of the ones I'd pressed, and it wasn't one of my better efforts. It was criss-crossed with a random pattern of creases. He picked it up with a look of horror. It had hardly been worn, but now it looked as though he'd been sleeping rough in it for the last six weeks.

He gasped, looked at his watch, threw me the venomous look that only a thwarted perfectionist can throw and ran off to do what he could with it in the five minutes remaining.

It seemed like a matter of only a few seconds before the door flew open. The sergeant stalked in, barked a few obscenities at us and ordered us to line up and show her what a bunch of rising stars we were.

'Come on, alphabetical order!' she shouted. 'As on the left, Zs on the right — or did mummy never teach you your ABC?'

We shuffled into position. As 'B' for Baldwin, I was second from the left next to — of course it was — Bucko. His shirt looked the way a paper pie bag looks when you've spread it out flat after it's been balled up in your pocket for a week.

We stood to some sort of attention. She advanced on Bucko, and then stopped short. She seemed momentarily lost for words.

'Well, I never!' screamed the sergeant, and then proceeded to give him a royal dressing-down for turning this all-important first inspection 'into a fucking circus'. I was chewing on the inside of my cheeks to stop from laughing. My mouth was full of the taste of blood and my eyes were full of tears.

Panting hard from all the shouting, the sergeant's eye passed over me and my un-ironed shirt. Off she went again, but she soon gave up on what she described as 'this farce'. If we didn't scrub up better by 0600 hours, she swore, there would be trouble.

There was a stunned silence after she left. Gathering the shreds of his heavily creased dignity around him, Bucko sloped off to his room for a bit of time out. Everyone began preparing for the next morning's inspection, but funnily enough, no one called on the services of their Chief Ironing Officer, even though, as always, I would have been happy to help.

It took a week or so for the whole notion of my being in the army now (or the air force, at any rate) to stop feeling surreal. Then I started enjoying it. The training was a mixture of classroom work, covering topics such as military law and history, along with a lot of physical training activities to ensure we were the lean, mean fighting machines that the nation needed us to be.

Rumour had it that officer cadets were traditionally given a hard time by the RNZAF NCOs who knew this was their one fleeting opportunity to give some shit to a bunch of people who would soon outrank them. All of us had heard much the same thing, but if anything, this shared belief worked in our favour. There was an unspoken agreement amongst us that we would present a united front if it came to it and it served to draw us together. I suppose it was a form of bullshit bullying, really, but in reflection it was all talk and I only directly experienced a couple of tense moments in my training.

On one occasion, while at the Combined Ranks Cafeteria, a large airman started butting his way in ahead of us in the food line as if he owned the place, but he responded to being pushed out again and was warned that a bunch of fives would follow his next attempt. Everyone knew that would have drawn the attention of the military police and that everyone would ultimately lose. Anyway, it seemed that after a period of time and the odd incident, it all settled down. Once you're in the military, whatever the rank, everyone feels the same family bond and takes good care of one another.

From what I could gather, the military has this belief that just about anyone with a normal IQ, in theory, can be taught how to lead others, and that once they're clued up, all that's needed to turn them into a General Patton or a Lord Nelson is lots of practice applying theory in the field. Obviously the military didn't want to waste time and money trying to train any man or woman off the street, so officer training candidates would be selected not only for their ability to learn quickly but also on the strength of some personal or psychological quality that suggested they had 'the right stuff'. That, of course, or a medical degree. They were pretty short of doctors when I applied.

What the military wants out of its leaders is people who know how to complete assigned tasks in the most efficient way using whatever is at hand in the way of personnel and resources. This meant we did a lot of group exercises, taking turns as group leader. As leader, you received a written set of instructions outlining what was to be done, how quickly it was to be achieved, and a list of the people and equipment available to you to complete the task. The exercises started out simple. We'd be given a couple of drums and a few planks and they'd ask us to use them to get our 'platoon' across an imaginary river. Each of us caught on to the rules of the game at different rates, but it wasn't long before we were acting, more or less, as a well-oiled team. This was just as well, because the tasks became increasingly complex and started to involve different skills, such as navigation and evasion tactics, all with the clock ticking on tighter and tighter timeframes.

Most of the time it went well, but I got into trouble once for clouting one of the troops who had done something annoying. I got a good old dressing-down from a couple of our teachers. In the middle of this lecture, our fun-loving padre took the heat out of the situation for me by throwing a live tear gas canister into the room we were in. ZING! We all flew out the windows like lightning as the acrid fumes billowed up. The padre wasn't popular with the bosses for this departure from standing orders. It made the little love-tap I had handed out look pretty insignificant. Thanks, padre.

It was generally known that our new-found teamwork and leadership skills would be put to a final test on a large-scale exercise in the foothills of the Southern Alps towards the end of the course. Besides exercising our highly polished officer skills, it would also involve lots of gear and some of the New Zealand military's most precious toys, like fighter jets and helicopters. We couldn't wait!

The day dawned cloudy and cold as our team — kitted out in camo gear, webbing and packs — was loaded up onto a bunch of big old army trucks. We were driven out and dropped off in the bush edge near Oxford Forest; just as we arrived, the cloud burned off and the sky shone that glorious, Canterbury shade of blue. We had to navigate our way to a set of coordinates deep in the mountains. If we could find the prearranged rendezvous point, we would then be picked up by RNZAF Huey helicopters and taken to 'safety'.

What made it extra exciting was that we were being chased by pursuing 'baddies' (or teaching staff pretending to be baddies) who would capture us if they caught us. There was also the slight risk of being hit by the Strikemaster jets that were carrying out a planned bombing run in the valley just before we were due to be lifted out by the choppers.

Bucko was the boss and I was the navigator: he eyed me, my compass and my obliging grin a bit warily. It all started well, but somehow we got a bit off-track and that really put us all under pressure. Fortunately I got us over a big ridge leading down into a wide river valley, and then downstream to the prearranged rendezvous point. This was amid the noise of the fast jets doing bombing runs up and down the valley, along with lots of yelling and screaming from the baddies in hot pursuit. Fun and games! I have to say that during this exercise I just couldn't believe I was being paid to do it. When the chopper finally lifted us out, I wanted to do it all over again.

Another memory I treasure from the IOTC was the lecture we received from a genuine, card-carrying war hero. The air force ensures that every intake of officer cadets is lectured by a veteran, and they take pretty good care to get someone who really knows what war is like. IOTC 889 was fortunate to have Wing Commander Johnny Checketts, DSO, DFC, talk to us. We were pretty excited when we heard, and we were all looking forward to it — a real-life commando coming to tell us his war stories.

Johnny was quite an unassuming bloke to look at and was getting on a bit (he was 77 at the time) but he was still in good shape. He was quietly spoken, and didn't have any flash audiovisual props to support his talk. But he had us spellbound. He told us about his first 'kill', a German ME-109 fighter over England. It wasn't quick or clean or impersonal: it all took place at close quarters, close enough that Johnny could see the terror in the eyes of the young German pilot as his plane caught fire around him, burning him to death in the cockpit. Johnny vomited and cried all the way back to base.

We stared at him, white-faced.

He reckoned the only thing that kept him fighting were the rumours that reached them from time to time about the atrocities that Hitler's Nazi arseholes were performing on the civilians of Europe. He was shot down twice; the second time he was quite badly burned. He was rescued and returned to England by the French Resistance. I didn't ever get the sense that he was proud of any of the death he dealt in the course of doing his duty. 'War is destruction,' he said. 'And that's not what human beings are here for.'

All of us, some more than others, probably had romantic notions of what it would be like fighting in a real war. Johnny pricked a few of those little bubbles. I reckon we all left feeling pretty lucky to have been born when and where we had, in peacetime in good old peace-loving New Zealand.

Massey agriculture graduates have a sort of a motto which goes: 'Two years ago I couldn't spell "farma" and now I are one!'

After four months of the IOTC, that's pretty much how Flt Lt D. E. Baldwin W93568 (Decorations for Bravery Pending) felt as he stood to attention in front of Wigram Airbase Museum to be presented with his 'You dun it good, son' certificate and — how awesome is this? — a sword. I was an officer! I was getting a sword, just like fucking Ivanhoe! When I marched out onto the parade ground, I had to fight the urge to forget this silly graduation parade and run out onto the runway and start chopping up all of the thistledown like I used to as a kid. Luckily, for the sake of my fledgling air force career, I didn't, and even though my dad had gone from this earth, I was sure he was sitting up there somewhere on a cloud, rapt that at least one of his kids had joined up and spent some time in the force he'd served for over 50 years.

Our warrant officer had a role to play in our graduation parade. He had scared the shit out of me when I first started the course, which probably meant he was doing his job. In the movies, fellas like him are hired to break the weakest new recruits because the brass don't want 'sissies' on the battlefield. In my opinion, no one gets the best out of a pupil by putting them under pressure with lots of yelling and screaming. As time wore on, we sort of got used to him bollocking on. But now here he was, all scrubbed up with lots of medals and shiny things hanging off the front of his uniform.

He approached me with my certificate; my awesome sword was laid out ready to be handed over on a velvet cushion at his elbow. He murmured his grudging congratulations through gritted teeth and extended his hand. I gripped it firmly. Got ya now, I thought, as his beady little eyes widened in shock. He glanced down, and — too late, because I now outranked him — he noticed that my apparently spotless white gloves were actually dotted with Twink, which had seemed the practical and easy way to paint out the marks and stains. I gave him a broad grin and garnished my firm handshake with a little tickle to his palm from my pinkie finger. It had the desired effect and he glared at me. I don't care if he thought I was a Freemason wanting him to join up or I was inviting him to share a gay old time together when our paths next crossed. Either way, it felt good to make my point.

You never broke me, you bastard.

Once the course was finished, I headed home to Palmy, but not for long. After two weeks' R&R, I reported for duty to RNZAF Base Ohakea, where I was shown to my new lodgings at the Base Hospital by the very officious chief administration officer who had the shiniest boots I had ever seen.

As we were well settled as a family in our Palmy lodgings, I was the first base medical officer (BMO) to live off the base. We had privacy that way, too, and it also meant we could keep all of the wonderful buddies who we'd grown to love during our early years in Palmy in our lives.

The BMO position involved five full days a week, with the need to stick around on the base when there was night flying in case of emergency. I also did a weekend on call with the local GPs. This seemed a real bind at first, but in retrospect, it kept me in tune with the outside community and introduced me to the GPs in Bulls, whose paths it seemed I was fated to cross.

The position of BMO called on me to wear two hats. One hat, of course, was that of the doctor who saw to the medical needs of base personnel. The other was my military hat; when I wore it, I was actually in command of a 'flight', which comprised 10 to 12 medics and the nursing officer who made up the staff of the Base Hospital. Being so well staffed, the hospital operated 24 hours a day and could offer quite a sophisticated level of care.

There were about a thousand or so staff serving on the base at Ohakea and many of them, along with their families, were accommodated on the base and in its immediate environs; it was my job as BMO to be their GP. This was the run-of-the-mill side of it, but I had the additional responsibility of keeping the operational staff — the aircrew, who were the pilots and navigators and engineers and so on, and the 'groundies', better known as the aircraft maintenance staff — fit for battle. So besides general practice, I was now a practitioner of 'occupational medicine' and, in particular, of 'aviation medicine'. Just as the aircraft maintenance personnel were in the business of keeping the planes airworthy, I was in the business of keeping both them and the aircrew fit for their purpose.

At Ohakea, I was dealing with aircrew who were flying high-performance aircraft that carried numerous objects that go 'bang', such as jet engines and ejector seats, not to mention a whole suite of nasty munitions. Quite apart from the obvious challenges to health and well-being posed by this, I was also dealing with people exposed to the stresses and strains that high-speed, high-altitude flying puts on the human body as a result of the G-forces, freezing-cold temperatures, low oxygen levels and low barometric pressure. Part of my job was carrying out regular medical examinations on all of the pilots and ensuring they were given first-class treatment if they got sick.

A good example of the way in which you need specialised knowledge when dealing with the aircrew of fast jets is the case of a young Australian F-18 Hornet pilot who I dealt with. He presented complaining of recurring, low-grade headaches at the back of his head. The flight operations he was carrying out involved circling around at 50,000 feet doing radar searches for 'enemy aircraft' flying at low level. If he detected any, he had to put his F-18 into a rapid descent to engage in simulated air-to-air combat with the enemy, routinely plunging 45,000 feet in less than a minute. After the combat session was over, he'd whizz back up to 50,000 feet in a minute flat. Then he'd do it all over again.

Whoa, I thought. Awesome.

Trouble was, his headaches were setting in during the rapid ascents and persisting while he was level at 50,000 feet. It was actually an easy diagnosis: sinus barotrauma.

Sinuses are gas-filled cavities behind your nose, and they are designed to cope with changes in pressure by allowing air to come in or air to flow out. If they're blocked, as this pilot's sinuses were, and you subject them to a rapid change in pressure (say, by flying to high altitude where the ambient air pressure is much lower), the pressurised gas in your sinuses compresses the surrounding tissue and causes pain: a headache. All it took to fix this pilot was a day on the ground to clear his blocked sinus passages using nasal sprays. A man or woman in the street would never really suffer from sinus barotrauma (unless they're into scuba diving); it's one of the joys of flying fast jets.

The pilots of jet-propelled warplanes are a special breed. They have to be. Modern fighter aircraft subject your body to a phenomenal amount of strain when they're under acceleration, or climbing steeply, or turning sharply, or spinning or diving, or any of the other things they have to do in combat situations. Pilots are expected not only to be able to endure this kind of carry-on, but also to monitor the highly complex systems that keep the plane flying and fighting at the same time. When you're locked in mortal combat with another aircraft in an F-18, or performing a tricky manoeuvre, such as refuelling a pair of A-4 Skyhawks at 20,000 feet above the Manawatu, you've got to have your wits about you. And even when you're just cruisin', the speed at which a life-and-death situation can arise when everyone who wants to jump you can travel at a couple of times the speed of sound means you still have to have your wits about you. The laws of natural selection see to it that not too many dozy jet-fighter pilots make it to a ripe old age.

The air force selects pilot officer cadets who not only have the necessary mental and physical toughness, but also are of the personality type that doesn't like to lose. I think the happiest I have ever seen a human being was on those occasions when a fighter pilot walked into the mess room after landing from one of their air-to-air combat training missions where they had got a 'fox one' or 'fox two' hit — a pretend missile impact — on one of their comrades. The flipside, of course, was the sick, gutted look on the face of their beaten opponent as he or she slunk off to the mission debrief. And it's not just in the air that this Type

A tendency surfaces; your average fighter pilot will die before he concedes defeat in any field of human endeavour, whether it's aerial combat, a day's fishing, a casual round of golf or how many Weet-Bix you can eat in a minute. Truth be told, it's pretty easy to mistake fighter pilots for out-and-out wankers. Yet I enjoyed just about every minute of working with this awesome bunch of men and women.

Like the pilots, the groundies are highly trained and have to be on top of their game, too, because of the complexity of the aircraft systems and also because of the danger. They routinely deal with high-pressure hydraulic systems, highly flammable fluids and gases, toxic chemicals — such as isocyanides — radiation-emitting electronics and all those dangerous munitions. One minor mistake could end in catastrophe. Mistakes occasionally happened, though thankfully nothing major on my watch. The worst was when an arrestor pin of some kind was placed in the wrong place in a jet's cannon. When the pilot went to do a pre-take-off systems check, he pressed the 'fire' button and a long volley of live 20-mm cannon-fire shredded the pasture in and around a herd of dairy cattle that was quietly chewing the cud. There was bedlam; over the next few weeks, milk production amongst the post-traumatic cattle dipped dramatically. It was a staunch test of the diplomatic skills of the Ohakea Base command, soothing the very pissed-off farmer!

Because of the peculiar demands of their job, I had to pay particular attention to the mental well-being of the groundies, too. All in all, my first taste of occupational medicine was a fascinating insight into the ways the role of a doctor can subtly differ depending on what their patient spends their time doing.

Of course, there were certain perks to being the sole BMO. Shortly after I took up my position, I managed to convince 75 Squadron boss John Bates that I really needed to have a ride in a fast jet, just so that I could get first-hand insight into the demands of that sort of aviation. So on 15 December 1989, I dressed up in a flight suit and donned a helmet and oxygen mask and climbed into the rear seat of the cramped cockpit of NZ6256, one of the New Zealand Defence Force's most prized possessions, an A-4 Skyhawk. The moment John lit her up and we hurtled down the runway, I knew that this was a bit of a step up from what I'd been flying around. The Kapiti coastline unrolled beneath us, and in a ridiculously short period of time, we were over Cook Strait. John dropped us to 50 feet and we skimmed along at 550 knots. If a kahawai had jumped, it was fish for breakfast. Just in case I hadn't really got the idea, John threw in a few aileron rolls for good measure — the sky and earth suddenly changed places and then flipped back again, all in less than a second as the plane spun on its axis. Luckily, I have a strong stomach; it was tight enough in the cockpit without sharing it with a bucket-load of chunder.

A little while after that first, unbelievable ride, I got wind of a forthcoming exercise featuring a four-ship strike mission: four A-4s flying in formation to their target, bombing the shit out of it and then returning. I indicated to John Bates that it would probably be a good idea, professionally speaking, if I got a taste of this kind of action, too, and he agreed.

I rode shotgun with Flight Officer Greg Elliott as we thundered off over the Central Plateau to the Bay of Plenty, tore out over the sea and really let the Volkner Rocks have it. The Volkners are a cluster of three small volcanic pinnacles just to the northwest of

White Island. I don't know what they had ever done to deserve it: perhaps some air vice-marshal had had a bad day's fishing out there or something, but they were a designated weapons-proving ground for the NZDF at the time. It was utterly fucking awesome! Sometime later, 75 Squadron organised a dinkum 'Fighter Doc' patch for me to wear on my flight suit and I must say that of all my qualifications, it's the one I hold most dear. It really made me feel part of the family.

I got to do all kinds of cool stuff, such as air-to-air refuelling of the A-4 Skyhawks at 20,000 feet surrounded by a beautiful sunset. Likewise, experiencing simulated air-to-air combat in an A-4 was an eye-opener; you get thrown around like a rag doll in the back of the jet due to the incredible G-forces involved in the ducking and diving needed to get the aircraft into position to 'shoot down' the adversary.

The older Strikemaster aircraft were fun to fly in because the two pilots were side by side, which made it easier to communicate. This meant when we were doing long cross-country trips around the North Island, you could have a right old conversation about various terrain features, or anything else that came to mind. The newly graduated pilots — or bograts, as they were called — loved taking people for a ride, as they didn't have a lot of responsibility and took any chance they could to build up hours. Often they'd be a bit naughty and do manoeuvres that weren't approved, like night-time aileron rolls. But if they were taking a slightly naughtier passenger along for the ride, who's telling?

The brand-new Aermacchis that turned up at Ohakea when I was the BMO were faster and more manoeuvrable, but unlike the Strikemaster, the pilots weren't side by side any more. The pilots were in line, one in front of the other. This made sense aerodynamically, because the jet was more sleek and rocket-like, but it just wasn't as much fun.

I flew in all of the other RNZAF aircraft that were stationed at the other bases: the Hercules, Andovers, Air Trainers and Iroquois helicopters. But the one aircraft I absolutely needed to do a full trip in was the four-engined Maritime Patrol Orions that were stationed at RNZAF Base Whenuapai near Auckland. I just loved these aircraft, and if I had been a general duties RNZAF pilot, they would have been my first choice. Getting to Whenuapai from Ohakea was easy in the RNZAF at the time; all I had to do was hitch a ride on a passing RNZAF Andover overnight and I'd be in the RNZAF Base Whenuapai officers' mess the next morning.

At Whenuapai I wandered up to the 5 Squadron hangar, had my emergency briefing and we headed off for an epic 12-hour flight to the Subantarctic. The first waypoint of the trip was buzzing the flight captain's mother's house in Timaru. We then carried on down to carry out supply drops to the workers on Campbell and Auckland islands. It was a great opportunity for me to see the Auckland Islands. I have always been fascinated by the many shipwrecks down that way — especially the *General Grant* in 1866 with its amazing survival story and the legend of all that lost gold.

It was hard to believe I was getting paid for this, along with the fact that I was getting first-hand aviation medicine experience of a kind that is now very hard to come by. Hey thanks, RNZAF.

CHAPTER 6

MY DESTINY IS IN BULLS

Ahhh, this is the life, I thought, as I touched our little two-seater Grumman aircraft down on Frank's Camden Farm airstrip located deep in the Awatere Valley of Marlborough. The aircraft rattled and shook as it taxied up by the shed, overloaded with guns, ammo, knives, binos, food and two very keen hunters.

'The goats are going to get it today!' exclaimed Marc excitedly as we stopped.

We jumped out of the aircraft and climbed straight into Frank's beat-up old Toyota Land Cruiser jeep. Frank was away mustering, but had thoughtfully left the jeep at our disposal. With a twist of the key it roared into life and we were off up the farm track heading towards an area we knew to be overrun by goats. Frank was very keen for private hunters to cull the goats, and we were very keen to oblige.

After 30 minutes of bumping and bone-shaking driving, we arrived at the end of the road and set off on foot to the crest of a sharp ridge that offers a great vantage point from which to glass the area for goats. We hadn't even gone 100 metres when beady-eyed Marc spotted three goats 60 metres away. Boom, boom, boom went the .223-calibre rifle and the job was done.

'Awesome shooting, Marc!' I said. 'You gonna leave some for me?'

'No way, Dad! I'm going to get them all.' His eyes were shining fit to make that big rock sitting on the top of the Queen of England's crown look like a bit of river stone.

Boy oh boy, I loved hunting with Marc. I had made a point of taking each of the kids out hunting as soon as I thought they were old enough, and while all three of them liked it, only Marc really got the bug. We went rabbit shooting anywhere we could find them in the Manawatu, and then, when I thought he was ready, we graduated to shooting at Frank's place in Marlborough.

=

After hunting, my passion was still flying. I decided in 1989 I would press on and get my commercial pilot's licence (CPL), which would enable me to fly passengers and freight for reward. Even if this didn't work out, I figured it would make me a better pilot. In those days Palmerston North was home to an outfit called United Aviation (which was no relation to United Airlines) that had grown out of the flying school set up by John Plank in 1994. A series of United instructors — Mike Hall, Simon Davidson and Garry Parata — guided me through the hoops. It was lucky for me that I was still in the RNZAF at the time because some of the RNZAF pilots pitched in to help, too, when they learned I was getting ready to sit for my CPL. I was having trouble holding a steady flight altitude and direction using only instruments in the civilian training aircraft, so I hitched a ride with John Bates to Whenuapai and got back in an A-4 Skyhawk at night so I could practise this technique. Not many budding commercial pilots these days can boast that they did some of their night-flying practice in an A-4 Skyhawk. I can tell you, it made an amazing difference to my instrument flying skills. Flying a fast jet travelling at 500 knots means you have to be very gentle on the controls; only the slightest bit of movement on the control column is required to change the jet's altitude, so sudden or large movements can get you into real trouble — like upside down when you don't want to be, or finding yourself all of a sudden a couple of thousand feet above your nominated altitude.

Likewise, my spin recovery was a bit dodgy, so a bloke called Topo took me up in an Air Trainer and put me through the ropes. Now these aircraft have a vicious and rapid spin which takes a bit of getting used to. Compared with the Air Trainer, a Cessna's spin seems like a walk in the park. In fact, you find you have to hold the Cessna's controls way over just to keep it in a spin; take your hands off the controls and it recovers by itself. Anyway, as with my instrument flying, the input of the RNZAF pilots helped me get my handling of spinning aircraft sorted. This, along with the good civilian training provided by Bob and co., got me through my CPL on 8 October 1990. My examiner was Ken Wells, who flew RNZAF Iroquois helicopters in Vietnam and received the Distinguished Flying Cross (DFC) for a particularly legendary piece of flying. Ken squeezed his chopper into a tiny clearing to extract several wounded men, all while the Viet Cong livened things up with guns and bombs. With that kind of nerve, he was a born flying examiner. He didn't scream once during my CPL exam.

'You'll do,' he said, at the end of the flight.

I completed my first commercial job just under a fortnight later, when a Dutch mate of mine hired me to take him up to photograph his farm. It was a short trip, but one neither of us will ever forget. I borrowed a mate's Cessna 172 that was based at a hangar on a farm near Marton. It was a beautiful Friday evening and I was pretty excited about the start of my career in commercial aviation. I skipped and whistled as I did the pre-flight checks. The plane's owner didn't have a dipstick to check the fuel level, but he assured me that if I could see fuel sloshing around level with a certain step in the tank visible through the filler cap, it was a third full. Based on this information, I satisfied myself that both tanks were a third full.

We loaded up and without further ado I cranked up the engine and off we went, heading south over Ohakea towards the farm in question. We did a few circles around it while my mate's camera clicked and whirred. Then it was time to head back to the strip at Marton. I thought I would make a quick detour to overfly Dr Bernard Lawson-Jones' house so that I could give him a wave.

Bernard was one of the local GPs who was to become a bit of a mentor to me when I started my medical practice at Bulls. He lived out in the sticks on a terrace just above the Rangitikei River.

MY DESTINY IS IN BULLS

I had tipped Dr Bernard off, and he was standing on the ground aiming a video camera at us. The first run over his house went well. We were just lining up for a second when that reassuring droning noise in front of us abruptly ceased. I was confused; I had plenty of fuel (or so I thought) and the engine had sounded fine right up until it stopped . . .

Still, there was no time to think it through.

Shit, I thought.

I might have said something along those lines, too, but I didn't panic. I just looked around for a paddock to crash-land into. I spotted one and began to line it up, but realised from the vertical airspeed indicator that we were falling from the sky faster than we were gaining on the paddock.

Ah, shit, I thought again, and might have said as much.

One of the things you're obliged to do for your private pilot's licence is demonstrate the ability to make a landing under simulated engine failure. This was not an exercise, but I managed to perform the manoeuvre — a side-slip and approach at full flap — to perfection, and lined up on another paddock. There were certain undesirable features in this paddock, but hell, beggars can't be choosers. The grass rushed up towards us, and we banged onto the ground.

So far, so good. We were still sunny-side up and in one piece.

We were going quite fast, and there was a bunch of very big poplar trees at the end of the paddock. I slammed on the brakes, pulling the stick hard back to try to get some extra weight on the wheels to slow us down. Meanwhile I aimed for a little gap I could see in the trees.

My mate had kept his composure remarkably well to this point, but now he suddenly burst forth in pidgin Dutch.

'Ach, der trees! Der trees! Vatch out for der fucken trees!'

I was curiously detached from it all, more fascinated by the way he had fallen between the stools of his native and adopted tongues than whether we'd live or die. I'd never heard him swear before, let alone speak Dutch.

We came to rest in the grove of poplars without having hit anything, and without having dropped into any of the deep holes that wallowing bulls had gouged in the paddock. We climbed out, shakily, and saw the farmer rushing towards us.

'What the fucking hell do you think you're doing?' yelled a rather red-faced Allan Willis, who owned the place. 'This isn't a bloody airstrip, you know!'

I explained the situation as diplomatically as I could to big Al, who eventually simmered down a bit. Of course, two decades later he still gives me stick about this episode every time I see him passing through Bulls. I think he's dined out on the story plenty; he even presented me with a framed picture of the aircraft after it crash-landed. It's hanging on the wall of the Bulls Medical Centre for all to see. And even if Al would let me forget it, there is a comprehensive video record of the whole sorry incident, courtesy of Dr Bernard, which is filed as 'Juiceless' in my archives.

Any aviation accident you walk away from teaches you valuable lessons. I shouldn't have flown this aircraft until the correct fuel dipstick was available. It was also all the excuse I needed to get my own aircraft, so that I could learn about it until I knew it backwards. Once home, and as soon as my nerves had settled down, I started looking.

MY DESTINY IS IN BULLS

=

Every year, 75 Squadron would fly its A-4 Skyhawks to a country in Southeast Asia to exercise with the combined sections of the Singaporean, Malaysian, Australian and Royal air forces and navies under the banner of 'Operation Vanguard'. Our A-4 Skyhawks were pretty old technology by 1991, but thanks to a blend of good old Kiwi cunning and ingenuity, they were still world class at both close-range air-to-air combat and maritime strikes (or blowing the shit out of ships).

When they weren't fighting on their terms, however, the A-4s couldn't match the F-18s and other more modern jets, because they had better radars and long-range air-to-air missiles that could take an A-4 out from 50 miles away. And the bugger of it is that the Australians had fully-loaded F-18s, which compounded any existing trans-Tasman rivalry and added to the already testosterone-charged business of supersonic jet fighting. Needless to say, short of actual war, this is what 75 Squadron's pumped-up jet jockeys lived for.

A huge amount of effort went into ensuring that we sent along a fully operational squadron performing at its absolute peak, and this in turn meant sending all sorts of elaborate equipment and numerous support personnel, including medical staff. In 1991, the medical support staff was me.

It was a seven-week deployment based at Kuantan, which is a large city on the eastern coast of Malaysia. I assured Sandi that it wasn't going to be a picnic. I painted a picture for her of the kind of accommodation I was expecting — a mosquito-infested, tented camp in a clearing hacked from tiger-haunted jungle next to a crocodile-ridden swamp. She set me up with lots of tropical-strength insect repellent and plenty of sunscreen, and I made sure I packed a spare boot to biff at the tarantulas.

The flight from Ohakea to Malaysia turned out to be a bit of a mission because it was Ramadan, the Islamic festival in which Muslims fast, pray, give to charity and neglect their air traffic control routines. This meant we had to fly right across Australia and way out into the Indian Ocean to the Cocos (Keeling) Islands in a massive dog-leg around Indonesia. The old RNZAF Boeing seemed to cope well, though, and no one in the squadron got too worked up about it. Of course, a beer in the Cocos Islands helped ease our sorrows.

When we finally arrived at Kuantan we were whisked to our not-so-rough quarters in the five-star Merlin Hotel. As unit medic, it was essential my room had the privacy necessary to conduct consultations with sick personnel. The concierge ushered me respectfully to a prime, beachside apartment that I had all to myself. I examined the patio and deckchairs and stole a glance at the panoramic view. There were Tigers about, all right: sitting there all dewy in the cool interior of the minibar.

'Will this do?' the concierge asked, and I nodded bravely.

That evening, reclining poolside with my third Fluffy Duck of the evening, I squinted at the dimming glow of the sunset over the South China Sea and reflected that training for war is hell.

We soon settled into a routine, which saw us scrubbed up in our uniforms, fed, watered and reporting ready for action at 0700 hours outside our hotel, from where we were driven to the Royal Malaysian Air Force Kuantan Airbase, about 20 kilometres away. The ground crews travelled by bus, but the pilots had a flash new air-conditioned minivan available to them so that they could come and go from the airfield at will. I usually tagged along with the pilots. Each day there was an arm-wrestle to see who got to drive — jet pilots like to be in control — but even though I love driving and did it professionally for a while, I was not considered.

Upon arrival at the airfield, the groundies and the aircrew would head off for their day of briefings and combat missions, while I would wander about doing bugger all. The local Malaysian base medical officer was a great guy, so I often popped over to have a very strong coffee with him. I also spent a lot of time getting to know the locals, who I enjoyed being with very much.

In the evenings, after a hard day's work winning the hearts and minds of the population, it would be back to the hotel for dinner and certain militarily essential cocktails. In seven weeks, I didn't do much actual medicine: besides a few mild cases of Delhi belly and a head cold or two, nothing much presented. But while it was a quiet time, it was also fun and bloody fascinating.

The Skyhawks did everyone — pilots, groundies, support staff and top gun doctor — proud. Occasionally you'd hear an Aussie F-18 or a Malaysian F-16 pilot having a big bloody boo-hoo about how the Kiwis were bending the rules of engagement and getting in close to kick their arses. That never failed to give me a surge of patriotic pride. But I also got a real appreciation of the wider value of these military exercises, too: the military, political and diplomatic mingling that went on really got New Zealand in there with these other countries, and won us a lot of admiration that aligned with the connections we had enjoyed since the Second World War. It wasn't long after this, in 2001, that the government, in a fit of short-sighted penny-pinching, dismantled and mothballed New Zealand's strike wing. They probably never realised how much damage they were doing to our international relations. Ah, well.

One day, in the middle of the exercise, the boys unanimously voted me driver for the day. I don't know what brought it about; perhaps they'd had too many Tigers the previous evening, which was a bit scary considering what they were about to do at the controls of supersonic aircraft in mortal combat. Or perhaps they wanted to spend the time in the back fine-tuning their tactics. I love driving: I didn't ask questions.

We set off on a beautiful Southeast Asian morning, with the sounds of happy yelling and arguing emanating from the A-4 pilots sat in the back. I weaved in and out of the bustling early morning traffic with a grin on my face, whistling now and again in between discussing the finer points of Malaysian cuisine with the very chatty young admin officer who was sitting up front with me. All seemed right with the world.

Suddenly, I spotted a dog lying in the middle of the opposite lane. It was moving, but it looked down and out; I assumed it had been hit by a car. If there's one thing I hate, it's to see animals suffer.

Without a second's hesitation, I swung the wheel to the right. There was a loud bang and shout from the back as the pilots were slammed against the left-hand wall of the van.

'Get over yourselves,' I muttered to myself. 'I'm on a mercy mission here.'

As we got closer, I realised the dog was bigger than I thought. In fact, I'm not sure I've ever seen a bigger dog. That was one thing. The other was that it was now showing every sign of being fully alert and perhaps not that badly injured after all.

'Shit,' I muttered, and the admin officer let fly with a blood-curdling scream as the dog's gaze met my own, a dawning awareness in its eyes.

There was a womp and a loud bong as the massive and quite agile animal disappeared beneath the vehicle, followed by another womp and a bong as the rear wheels went over the poor thing in their turn. The second noise was accompanied by various thumps and bangs and loud screams from the pilots.

Every imaginable form of motorised transport was now speeding towards me — buses, rickshaws, vans, trucks, cars . . .

'Fuck,' I muttered, swinging the wheel hard to port and then just as hard to starboard to regain my own lane. The pilots, flung right and left, roared their disapproval, and the admin officer sobbed quietly in terror and confusion.

I heaved a sigh of relief, but it was premature. While the van had resumed business as usual, flying straight and level at 80 km/h on the correct side of the road, I had over a dozen bruised and angry pilots to answer to, not to mention the poor admin officer. She had been homesick enough before she climbed in the van with a madman who murdered an innocent creature that bore more than a passing resemblance to her own beloved pooch back in New Zealand. I tried to tell everyone that I was only doing the decent thing and putting a poor, defenceless mutt out of its misery, but no one seemed inclined to listen. My name was mud for a few days, and I sure as hell didn't get to drive the van again.

Back in New Zealand, in mid-1991, after all the fun and games of Operation Vanguard, I reflected that I had been in the RNZAF for nearly half of my three-year contract. The RNZAF was offering plenty of incentives to stay on: at the end of my term I would be entitled to go on an 18-month study leave-of-absence overseas with Sandi and the kids, all expenses paid. They invited me to do a wings course, which would see me qualified to fly strike aircraft, and guaranteed me a tour of duty in 75 Squadron flying A-4s. And what's more, I wouldn't have to stay on much longer to qualify for the generous serviceman's pension, too.

The wings course was very tempting, but it was long and intensive and would mean another lengthy stint away from Sandi and the kids. And the trouble with the military as a career is that you have no say over where you'll be deployed and when; the life of the kids of soldiers, sailors and airmen is one of constant moving from place to place and school to school. Neither Sandi nor I wanted that for ours, who were pretty well dug in to the school and community in Palmy. The pair of us enjoyed the circle of friends we had locally, too, and there were our extended families to consider.

So it was time to rethink my career direction again and luckily there was an option sitting right in front of me.

Soon after I had started at the Ohakea base, I had paid a courtesy call to the local GP practice in the quaint little town located just across the Rangitikei River. Bulls is the only town of that name in the world, although it does have a sister town, of a kind, called Cowes on the Isle of Wight in the UK. The (New Zealand) town's name derives from its founder, Mr James Bull, who established it after setting up the general store in 1859. In its early years, the town had a variety of names: Killeymoon, Taumaki, Bulltown and Rangitikei. But as James Bull owned and controlled just about everything in the developing town, the locals simply referred to it as Bull's. In 1872, Bulls shed its apostrophe and became official. Its uniqueness was proudly exploited by one of its illustrious citizens, Major Wilson, who served in France and Belgium during the First World War. He simply addressed telegrams he wrote to his mother: 'Mrs Wilson of Bulls'. Even though he gave no further information — not even naming New Zealand as the destination country — they always arrived on time and at the correct address!

The town was situated where it is because of its strategic location next to the Rangitikei River, which in the pioneer days allowed for easy access inland from the coast. Later, Bulls became an important State Highway 1 crossroads, joining the main highways of the North Island, so the town has always done well out of the business that travellers bring with them. These days Bulls has a population of about 2000 people in the town and another 2000 in its rural hinterland.

The general practice started in 1900 with the arrival of Dr Watson, who worked in Bulls until his retirement in 1946. Doctors Geoff and Joan Walton took it over in 1947, which meant that when I met them, they had been practising for the better part of 50 years. After all that time, they made no secret of the fact that they were ready to move on. Indeed, if an investment they'd made in a kiwifruit orchard over in the Bay of Plenty hadn't come a gutser, they would have been out of there already.

When I first walked into their practice rooms — an unassuming little house on High Street — I might as well have been on a different planet, because not only did the equipment belong in a museum, but patients were handled in a very old-school way, too. I showed up punctually at ten o'clock, just in time to hear Dr Geoff's old grandfather clock strike the hour. The grandfather clock was synchronised to the atomic clock in Zurich, and tea and scones were served by the nurses at 1000 hours precisely, when everything ground to a halt.

The consulting room door was half open as I was walking past that morning and I saw a patient dutifully nodding as Dr Geoff stood up, gave a half-hearted wave and without a word left the room for his mid-morning sustenance. The patient waited meekly for his return in a very quiet and dark consultation room for the next 15 minutes without saying dickybird. That was the way it went.

Similarly, a long-time patient of the practice recently asked me, just after I had taken his blood pressure, what the reading was. I told him, '120/70'. The patient told me that when he had politely asked the same question of Dr Walton a few years ago, Dr Geoff had haughtily replied: 'It's not your right to know.' That's the way medicine was back in the day, but thank goodness things have changed. I suppose I should be grateful, though, because when I bought into the practice, it came with a full stable of very well-trained patients.

In my opinion Dr Geoff and Dr Joan did an outstanding job working as the sole GPs in the area for so long. It's easy to forget how hard it would have been to be a country doctor in the late 1940s through to the 1960s, what with the isolation and being on call 24 hours, seven days a week. I was pleased to see that after their retirement, they both received the Queen's Service Medal for the good work they did for the community. Having taken over from them by then and seen first-hand what they dealt with, I think they should have received knighthoods.

In 1991, just after I got back from Malaysia, Geoff Walton asked me whether I would like to buy the practice. I declined at the time, but it did get me thinking. The Waltons' practice was still the only GP service in an area extending from Marton to Turakina Beach out west, down to Rongotea, just south of the airbase at Ohakea, and further south still to Himatangi, so it had huge potential. I talked it over with Sandi, and it all seemed to fit: we would keep our proximity to our friends, family and school community in the Manawatu, not to mention the Tararuas, and if all went well, it was a return to The Jacobsen Plan. I could divide my time between doctoring and my other loves: I could have my cake and eat it, too.

So I took the plunge, tendered my resignation papers to Her Majesty and signed up the purchase agreement, which gave me full ownership of the Waltons' general practice in Bulls. They helped me hang up my shingle, and it was a very proud moment to step back and see it there. I was quite sure I had done the right thing.

I started consulting for the first time on 8 May 1991 at their old rooms, which I leased from them under the trading name of 'Bulls Medical Centre Ltd'. On the surface, it might have seemed silly using this name, when the practice only comprised one dodgy doctor (me), three part-time nurses (Julie, Julie and Judith), one admino (Elaine) and a rowdy cat (Bob). But the name Bulls Medical Centre Ltd kept me motivated to develop the potential of the practice and I hoped the small band of thieves that we were could one day grow into a true medical centre, and one that would make the region proud.

It wasn't going to happen by itself, but I wasn't scared. Now that I was out of the protective environment of the RNZAF, and had become a self-employed solo rural GP, it was time for head down and arse up. I've never been afraid of hard work.

A few months after this latest, life-changing career move, I took steps towards realising the dream of owning my own aircraft, too. I had sounded out the Powers That Be at Ohakea Airbase and had received permission to hangar a light plane on base, and by then I thought I had tracked down a suitable plane, too. On 26 September 1991, Sandi, Niki and I drove to Pine Park airfield just outside Foxton to catch up with our old mate Richard Scott, Pine Park's co-owner, who had a Grumman AA-1B two-seater T-Cat for sale, registered ZK-DNI. The T-Cat is a little low-wing affair — which means the wings are mounted under the cockpit rather than slung over it, as in the high-wing Cessna — and it seats two in a cockpit that you get into by sliding back the Perspex canopy. That makes it feel a bit like a Second World War fighter, and what's not to like about that? Richard checked me out on ZK-DNI, then I took both Niki and Sandi up for trial flights. We all finished up with great big grins on our faces, so I paid Richard the big bucks and ZK-DNI — soon to be known as 'ZK-Doctor-Never-In' — was all ours. It was a great thrill flying our first aircraft from Foxton to its new home at RNZAF Base Ohakea.

MY DESTINY IS IN BULLS

Now that I was master of my own domain, I was free to do some commercial VFR (visual flight rules, where you fly by instruments and without visual reference to the ground) work for United Aviation. The company had started taking small groups of couples for joyrides around Palmerston North in a Piper PA-32 Cherokee Six. They would turn up in a limousine looking all shipshape in their finest duds, go for a romantic flight above the dazzling night-time spectacle that was Palmy and then head off in the limo again for dinner. It sounded awesome, provided the pilot was good at night landings as opposed to collisions of aircraft with ground.

My first gig went like clockwork, at first. The limo glided up and the driver, who was all done up in a dorky uniform, opened the back door and ushered the two unsuspecting couples over to the ready-and-waiting aircraft. I greeted them and got them seated, set up the dorky-looking driver in the co-pilot's seat, settled in myself and then started up the aircraft. The driver decided to give a running commentary as I taxied to the runway, took off and then cruised around Palmerston North, which was gloriously lit up by a full moon. To listen to him, you'd think he was an ex-fighter pilot and knew everything about flying. It got quite irritating. Thankfully, it was only a short flight; after five minutes of circling, I descended into the landing pattern and lined up on runway 07 for landing.

Up to this point, I had struggled with night landings. I tended to flare the aircraft too early — lifting the nose to reduce the speed of descent. I was concentrating on not doing it this time around.

'Now he's lining up on the runway. Shortly he'll flare up,' the driver said smoothly, not noticing I had already flared up. 'I reckon she'll just grease on in.'

Instead, we dropped the last 20 feet like a stone and banged into the runway. The passengers shrieked as the aircraft bounced a couple of times.

'Well, you got that one wrong!' I told the driver. He was so shaken by the uncalled-for bump on his bum that he turned all pasty and didn't utter another word. In fact, an awkward silence prevailed during the taxi back to the limo; I didn't even have to help them out. The aircraft doors burst open and they bolted out to the waiting limo without even saying goodbye. Ungrateful buggers, I thought.

CHAPTER 7
FREEDOM IS COMING

The dream had always been to combine the things I love and, by the end of the 1990s, it was all beginning to come together. I had always admired the free-spirited people who flew choppers around the Southern Alps for a living, ever since I had first come into contact with them. Dave Saxton and his son Morgan typified this special breed.

Since I first met Dave while working for the Forest Service towards the end of 1977, he had moved over to the West Coast to set up shop in Haast, where his legend had continued. Dave was very similar to Mum in that they came alive in the bush and the mountains. If you only knew them in the confusing, civilised world of towns and modern appliances, you didn't really know them at all. In the wild blue yonder of the Southern Alps, they became beautiful beings who were at one with the environment. Granny Olive would disappear into the bush and you'd hear her singing with the tuis as she fossicked around the forest floor looking for unusual herbs or orchids. Dave, on the other hand, would make a beeline for the cliffs or riverbeds to examine the rocks for signs of gemstones or pounamu. When he found something of significance, his rough hands would caress the stone as gently as if it were a lover's thigh.

Morgan, Dave's eldest, had grown into a big, strong kauri tree of a man with a smile as broad as the Haast River mouth. He was more at home with the toys of modern-day *Homo sapiens*: he just loved his Hughes 500D and spent long periods of time tidying it up and polishing the windscreen between flights. Morgie had also become a legend in his own right. I used to watch Dave and Morgan together as father and son and reflect on how cool it must be to be part of such a great team. I thought maybe Marc and I could have some of that action; now that he was nine, I figured it was high time he got a glimpse of this side of New Zealand.

In April 1998 Dr Pete Morrison joined the Gang of Three — Granny Olive, Marc and me — and we flew to Haast in a hired Cessna 182 with our hunting and camping gear.

Morgie Saxton flew us to Creswicke Flat Hut in the Landsborough River valley. This was our first real trip together into the wild Southern Alps. With his curly dark hair and his almost Baldwin-esque good looks, Morgie was on great form and Marc just lapped up all his bullshit. Marc had been up in my brother Andrew's helicopter a few times, and had probably already started to dream of a career in choppers. But this flight up into the magnificent landscape of Fiordland, as well as many other flights with Morgan, surely cemented the dream.

If Marc was impressed by Morgie, he was positively gobsmacked by the awesome spectacle of a wild, untamed animal in its natural habitat. I refer, of course, to Granny Olive, who really came alive in the outdoors. She grew up in the mountains, spending many of the best times of her life not far from where we camped. She could point at the majestic summits of some of the highest peaks surrounding us and proudly say: 'Climbed that. Stood there.' You simply couldn't find someone who loved being in that environment more than Granny Olive.

On this and subsequent trips, we would select our campsites so that Mum could look up from her duties as camp mother and rest her gaze on the mountaintops. Her knowledge of the natural history of her surroundings was incredible. If it moved, she knew what it was. If it didn't, she knew what it was, too. Animal, vegetable or mineral, the entire landscape was like an old friend to her.

She herself, though, wasn't so easily identified or categorised. In hot weather, she had no qualms about stripping down to her rather unsightly bra and pants, and she would move about the camp humming happily to herself in this state of advanced undress.

'Granny Olive,' Marc asked once. 'Do you know you've got a hole in your undies?'

'Oh, yes,' she replied cheerfully. 'That's just to let the gas out, dear.'

You'd think she was unaware there was anything odd about the way she dressed, but of course, she knew. She just didn't care, and we loved her for it.

On that 1998 trip, we were in the Creswicke Flat area for eight days, hunting up the spurs to where the bush gives way to the alpine tussock. Just to the south of the hut there's a huge fan of wide open bush running directly off the steep mountainsides, and it's ideal country for deerstalking.

Marc and I were working our way up an old, dry riverbed that was criss-crossed with deer trails. From the top, we had a grand view of the bushland to the south. We sat down to glass it, and couldn't help noticing a couple of odd-looking ponga logs lying in a gap between a bunch of trees. I put the telescopic sight on them, trying to work them out.

I handed the rifle to Marc.

'Do ponga logs breathe, Dad?' he whispered.

'What?' I exclaimed, and after another look with the scope magnification wound up fully to 9x, I saw he was right. The so-called logs seemed to be slowly moving up and down as if they were breathing. And as if to banish any last doubts, one of the 'logs' rolled over and stood up, revealing itself to be a rather sleepy young stag.

'Get it!' squawked Marc, as if I needed any encouragement.

I placed a .270 round directly into its chest and, just like that, we had claimed our first deer together as a team. It was such a buzz. We kept talking about it as we skinned the beast out, and as we walked back to the hut and then again after dinner and well into the night. Of course, by this time, we had improved on a few details of the story, as hunters always do: the bush was thicker, the range was greater, the wind was stronger and the beast was pawing the ground and full of aggro . . . It's all part of the fun.

While we were passing through Haast, Dave Saxton asked me whether I would do an aviation medical for a mate of his. Pilots are obliged to have regular medical examinations, with the examiner providing a certificate to the Civil Aviation Authority to confirm that the pilot isn't a danger to themselves or others, medically speaking. Inspections get more frequent the older you are, and the older you are the more likely you are to develop a condition, as the rules put it, 'of aeronautical significance'. In 1991, I had flown down to Paraparaumu to do a few of these for my brother Richard, who had his own aviation training company called Welair, and I was happy to oblige Dave Sax and his mate, too. It occurred to me afterwards that if I got enough of these examinations lined up in the nation's pleasure spots, I could get other pilots to pay for my trips around the countryside. How cool would that be?

Back in Bulls, I was head down and bum up in the medical centre on the afternoon of 5 May when one of the staff told me that there was a policeman wanting to see me.

'There's been a crash involving your brother Andrew's helicopter,' he said.

Wow. It's amazing how a one-liner can make you freeze. It felt like a kick in the guts.

'Is he OK?' I asked, but somehow I knew the answer. Even

when he told me that there were three people involved and that two were dead, one alive, I just knew. We screamed around to his house but he wasn't there, and we couldn't get him on the phone. Soon, we got news that there had been a mistake. There were only two people involved in the crash, and both were dead.

What seemed to make it worse was that Andrew had been dragging himself out of a bit of a hole. His first marriage had failed a year or two before, and he went through a pretty bad patch for a while. He had been a professional firefighter when, to everyone's surprise, he had reinvented himself as a chopper pilot. It blew us all away, as he'd never really expressed any interest in flying before, but when he put his mind to it, the commercial helicopter pilot licence came quickly — another example of how personal achievements are possible when you're really determined to make it happen. He'd also met and married his second wife, Josie, and it looked as though he was on the mend.

According to Mum, Andrew had phoned her that morning to say that he was going to do a little freebie for a mate of his in the foothills of the Tararuas, inland from Waikanae. He was lifting ponga logs out of the bush using a sling on a 40-foot line beneath his Hughes 300. What seems to have happened is that the sling snagged momentarily, and because he was using a 20-odd-foot rope in combination with his usual 22-foot lifting chain, the elasticity of the rope caused the chain to whip up into the main rotor. Even though the machine wasn't that high off the ground, there was no chance of surviving the tremendous forces that were unleashed when the rotor blades disintegrated.

Andrew's death hit us all pretty hard, especially Mum. It was a difficult time for everyone.

Marc and Andrew both walked with a stoop, like helicopter pilots, as though avoiding the rotors. They also shared a mannerism: when they were amused by something, they'd both smirk crookedly, duck their head and look away. Whenever Marc did it, I would be hit with a pang of both love and loss.

=

Meanwhile, the Bulls Medical Centre was trucking along. I had no problem dealing with the long trail of patients suffering from every type of pestilence imaginable, but the administration was getting out of hand. I had been toying with the idea of getting a manager for a while when Karen Greer turned up for a consultation. She seemed to be pretty competent and was looking for a job, so I asked a few questions to suss her out, such as: 'Can you make fruitcakes?' and 'What about typing?' Her answers were satisfactory, so I surprised her by offering her a job.

'Doing what?' she asked.

'I don't know,' I shrugged. 'I suppose you could start by maybe trying to manage this zoo.'

A day or so later, I had a manager and she was, and still is, an amazing worker. However, like all people, she's not perfect. For example, medical transcription is a highly specialised branch of the secretarial arts, and she didn't master it at once. One day she typed up a letter I had dictated to a surgeon about a patient who was suffering from 'intermittent claudication', which is a form of blockage of the arteries. However, instead of claudication, she wrote 'this patient is suffering from intermittent fornication'. You can imagine the smart reply I got back from the surgeon, who felt that he'd be acting well beyond his professional expertise in trying to deal with this one.

My old buddy Chris Williams was an orthopaedic surgeon by now, and had moved to Palmy to set up shop. We were very lucky, as he included a couple of clinics a month with us at the medical centre, which was a marvellous service. I also built solid working relationships with other GPs, including Dr Ruth Carter, who lived locally on a farm. Dr Ruth started by working one full day a week and then built it up to a few days. Working with another GP on the premises took a bit of getting used to, but Dr Ruth was such a help and was always available to give advice. I am and always have been a lone wolf, but Dr Ruth convinced me that there are advantages to working with a pack from time to time.

I started annually recruiting GP trainees to work with me for a complete year — a longer experience for them but a broadly similar one to my stint at Fiordland back in the day — which would see them through to the completion of their GP exam. This worked out really well; I found it stimulating to have younger doctors around. And it was very constructive both for me and for the practice, more than offsetting the extra work required to provide training and supervision.

All the same, I wasn't ready to share the practice with anybody yet. I had seen a few practices bust up because of doctor incompatibility, and I took the rather selfish view that, even though I was working way too hard, the Bulls Medical Centre was my baby with a certain loose, happy atmosphere. I feared that if I had a business partner, they might turn out not to be my type —

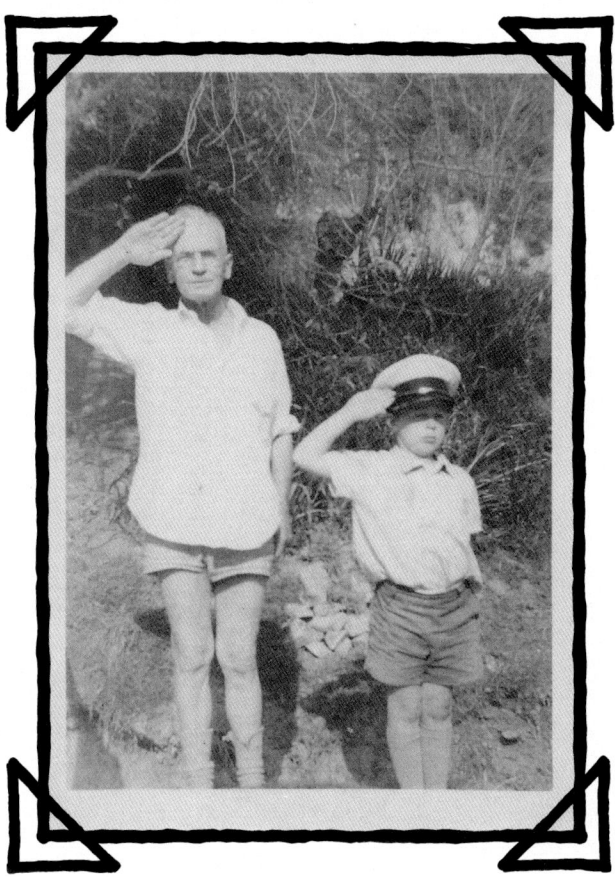

Good old Dad loved to play military games with me
— Colonel Dave and Sergeant Dad!

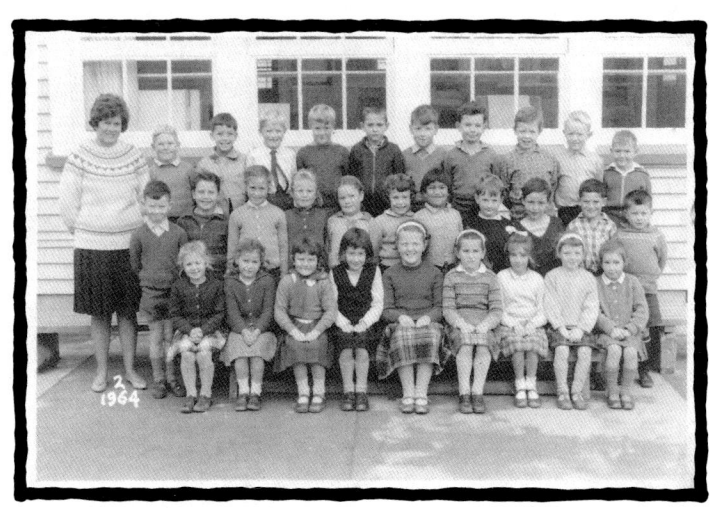

Me and a few of my scallywag mates at Paremata School in 1964.
(I'm in the top row, third from right.)

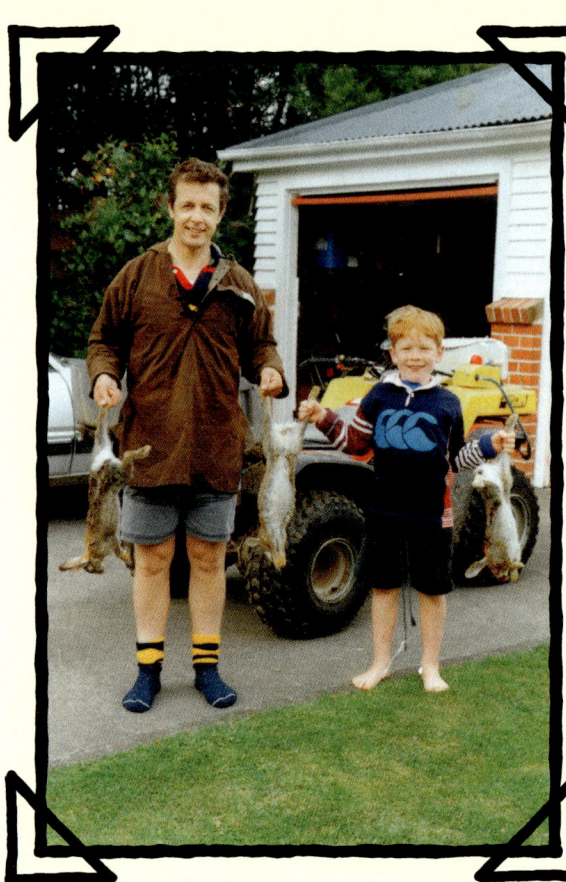

A good morning's hunting with Marc, the young hunter in training.

Granny Olive ready for action near the Gorge River, 1991. The knife she wore was for defence against any wayward stags that might confront her.

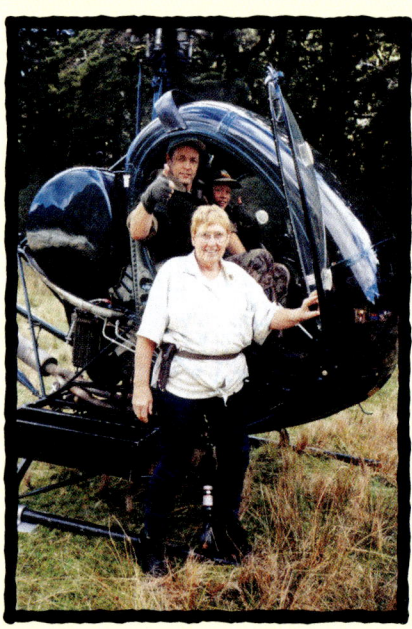

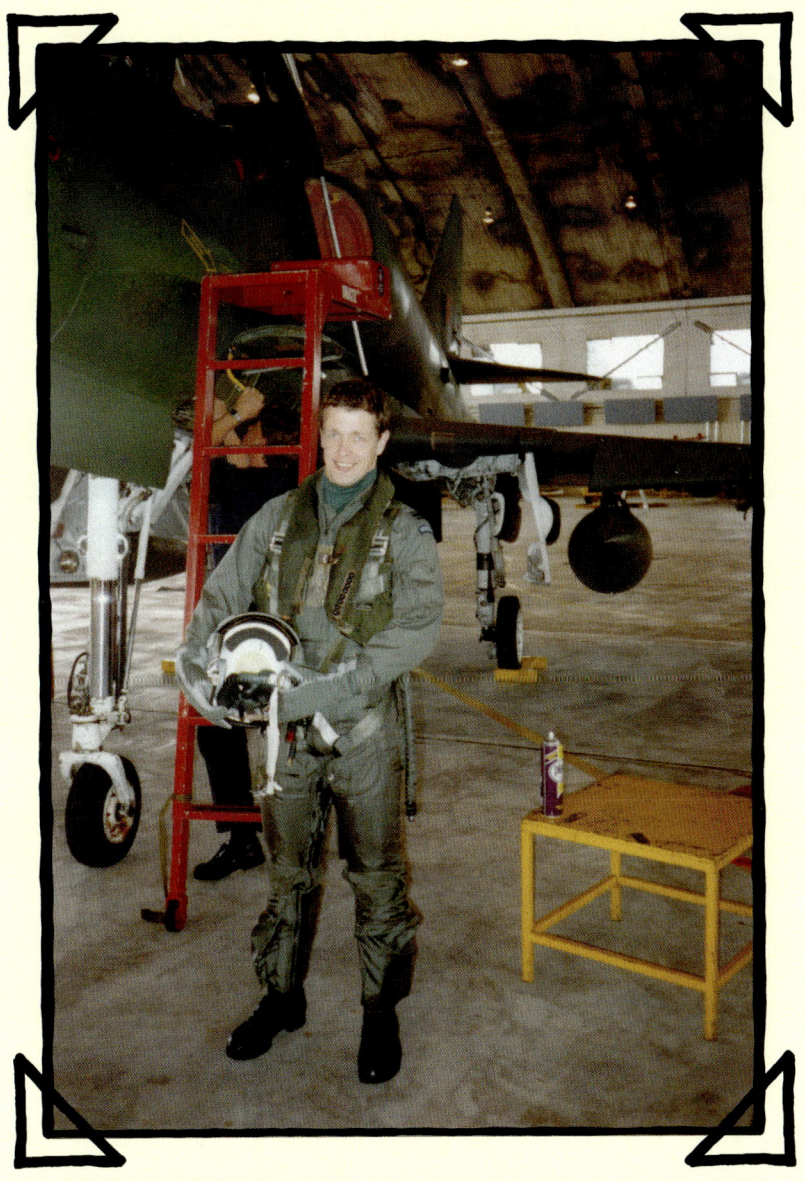

The RNZAF Base Ohakea gave me the most amazing practical experience in aviation medicine, as well as lots of rides in fast jet fighters.

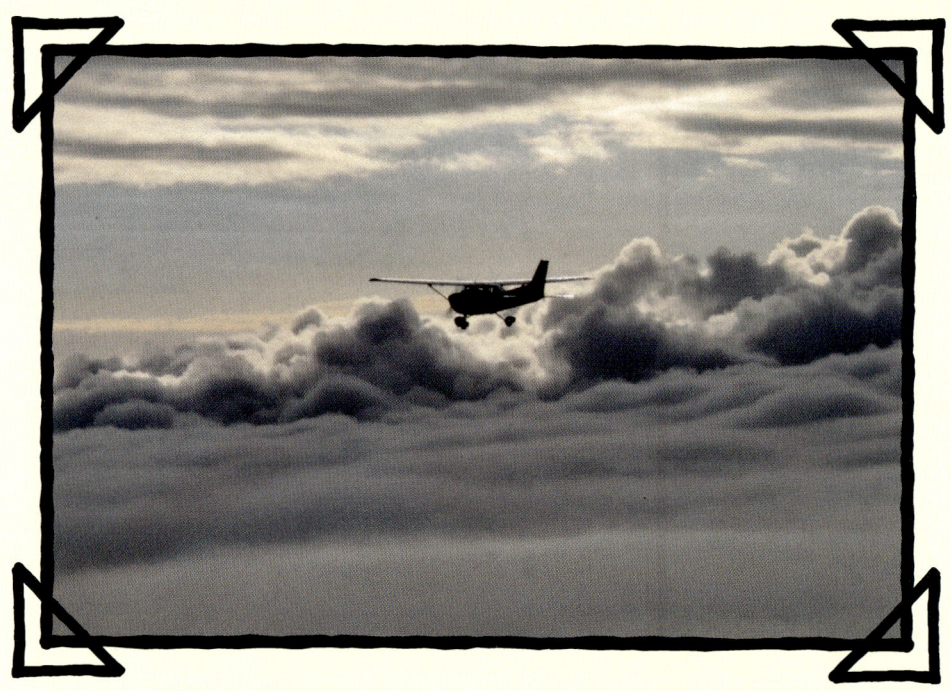

ZK-Really-Jolly-Good heading into the Deep South on one of my flying doctor rounds.

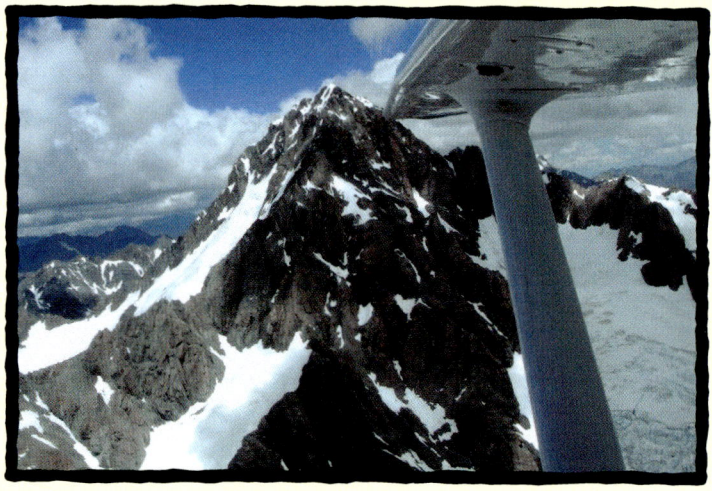

Mount D'Archiac just off the wing tip deep in the Southern Alps — now this is flying!

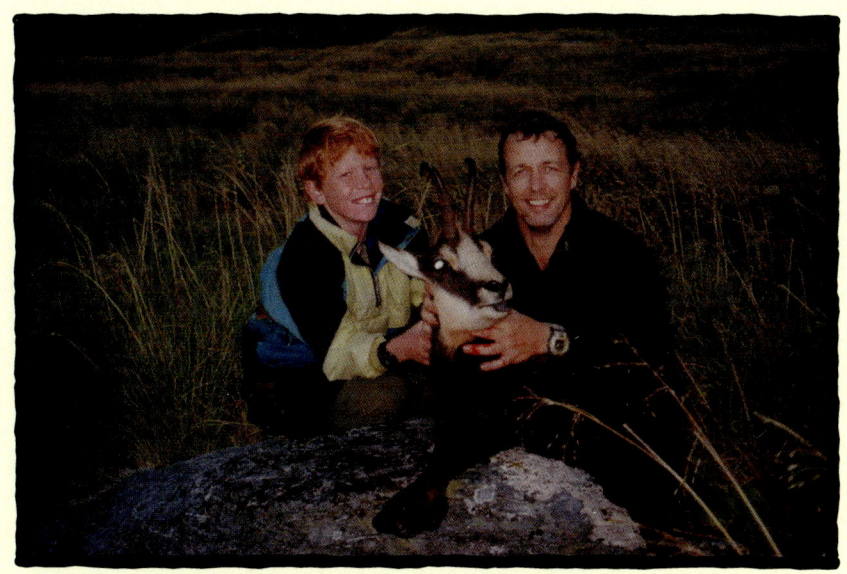

Another chamois hits the dust thanks to Marc's sharp shooting.

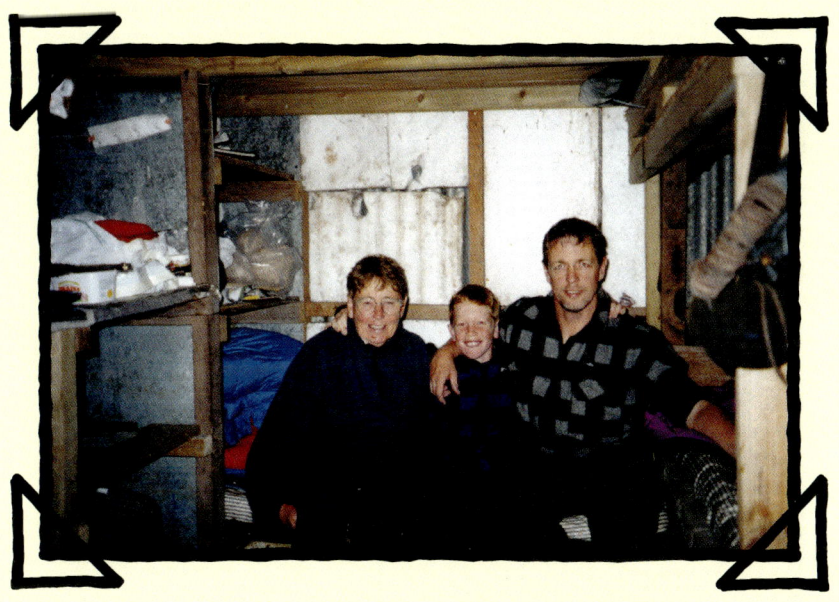

The Gang of Three: Mum, me and Marc having good times at the old Fraser Hut in Landsborough Valley, South Westland.

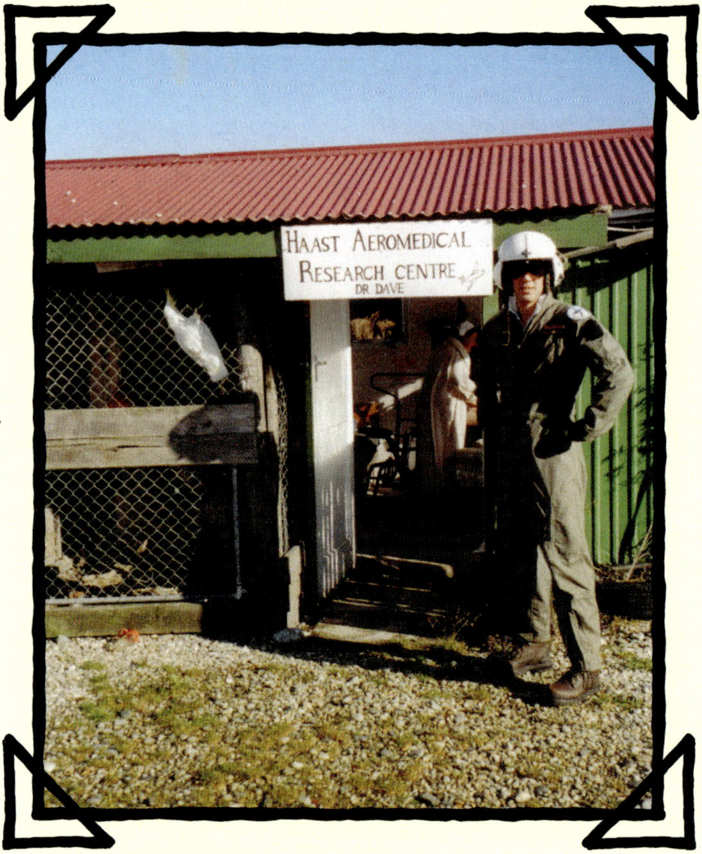

Morgan Saxton dressed as the fast jet pilot he was, standing next to the ill-fated parrot — the gate guard of the first Not-So-Royal Bulls Flying Doctor Service (NSRBFDS) outpost in Haast.

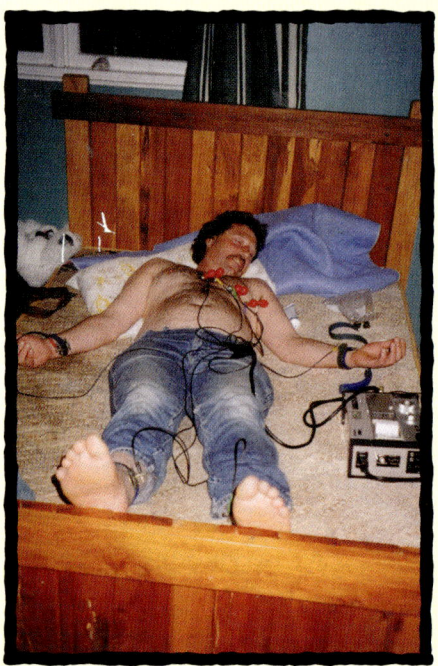

Harvey gets an ECG in the early days of the NSRBFDS in Haast.

Dr Malcolm Abernethy prepares himself for the mother of all hunting trips with me, my dog Camellia and I.

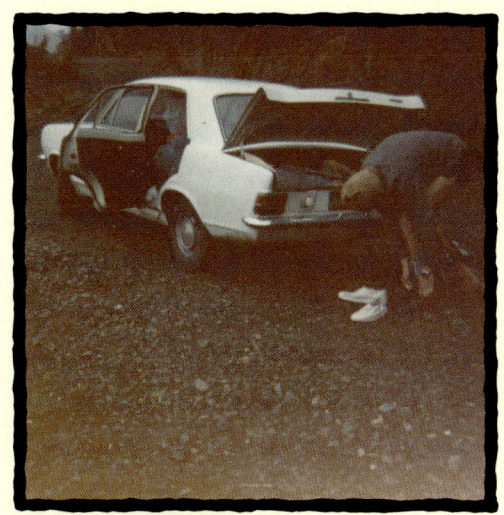

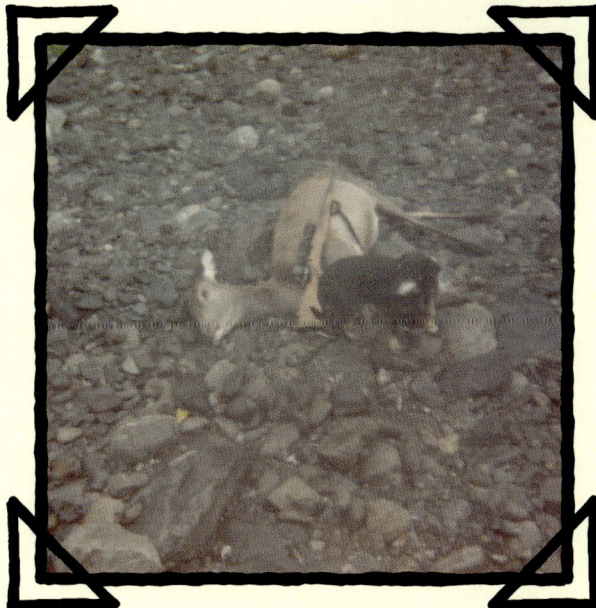

Camellia, the ultimate deer-tracking hound in the West!

Dr Malcolm's relationship began badly with this happy hound, but he ended up sleeping with her.

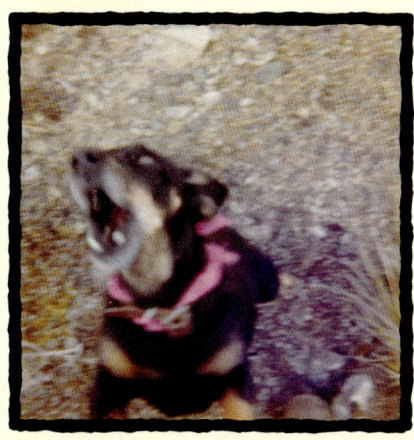

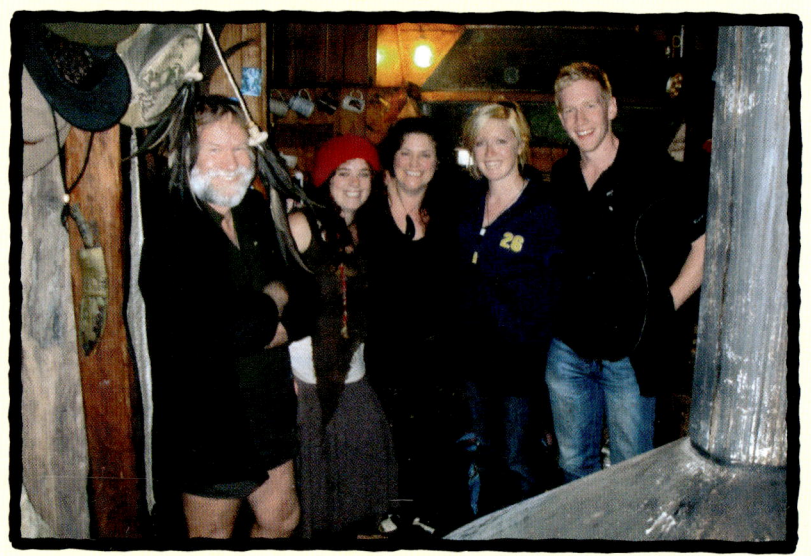

The awesome Salters at Pukekura with Marc and Niki — what great people!

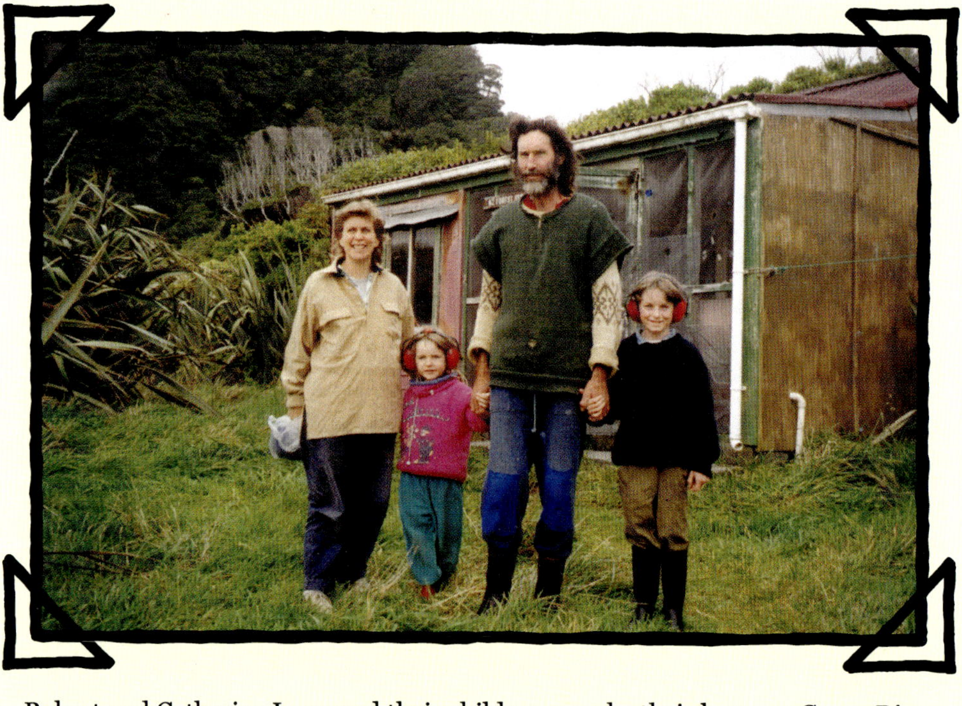

Robert and Catherine Long and their children pose by their home at Gorge River.

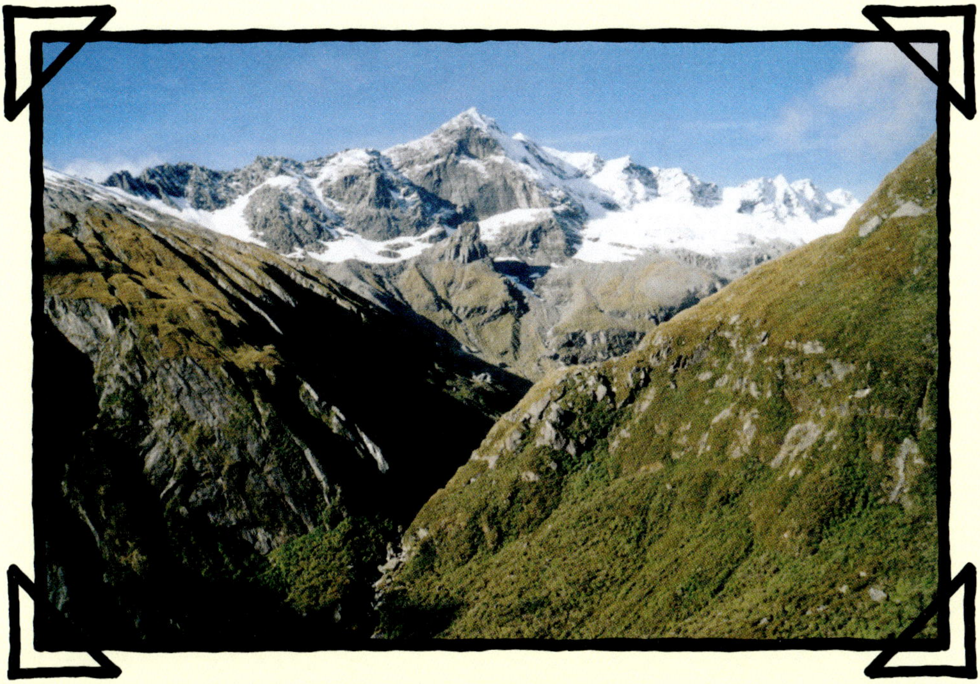

The big mountains of the Southern Alps are the ultimate playground for the free spirits of this country.

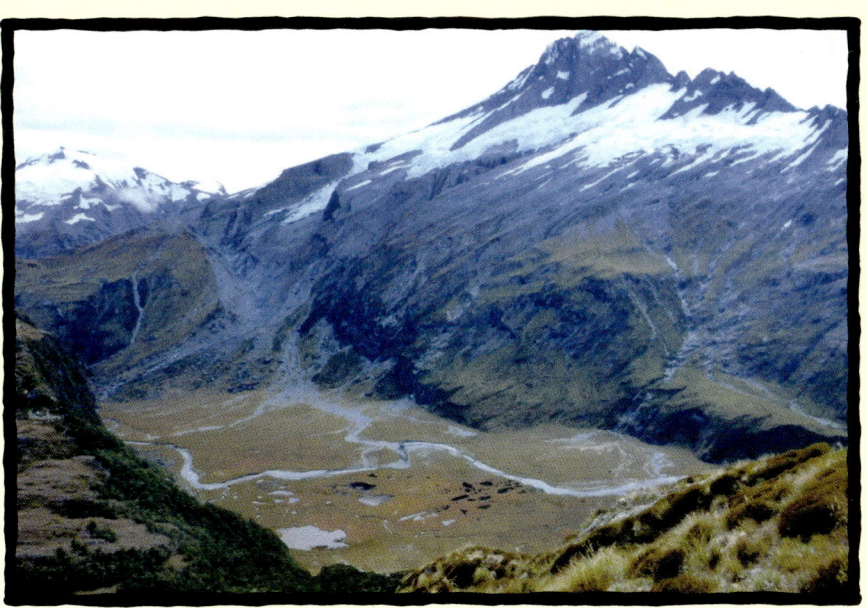

Marks Flat under the mighty Mount Hooker, located deep in the South Westland mountains.

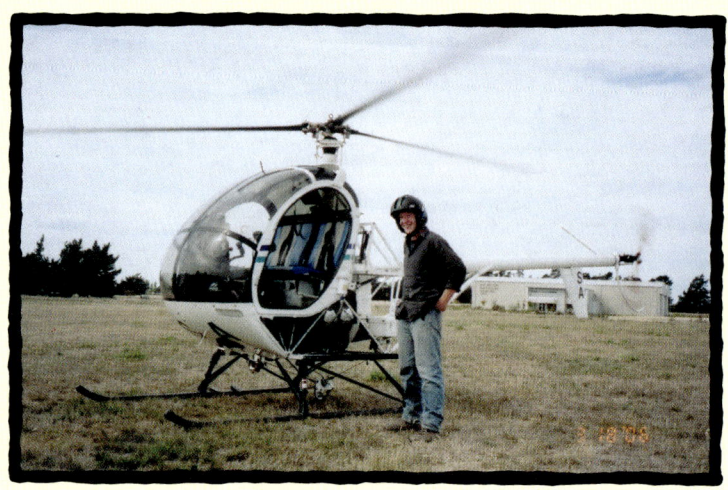

Chopper pilot Marc with a grin the size of the Ganges River — the dream is a-happening!

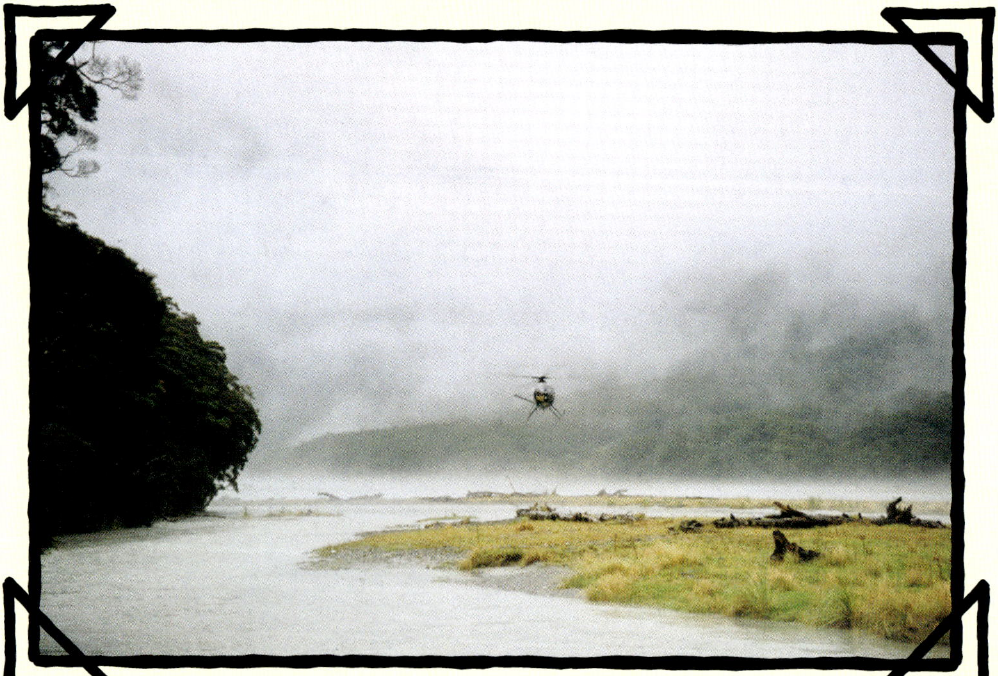

The Waiatoto River, South Westland, in full flood due to heavy rain that only West Coasters know.

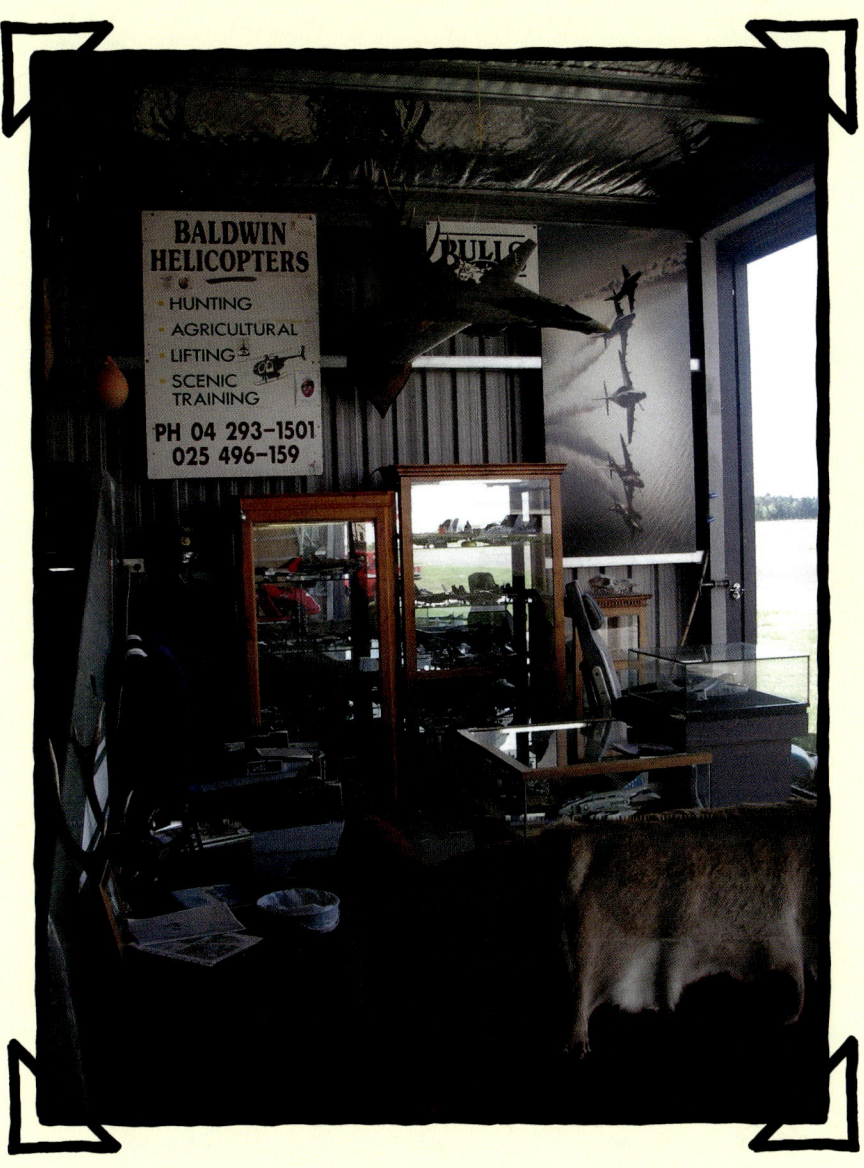

A smoko room like no other, with an awesome view of the airstrip, at NSRBFDS headquarters.

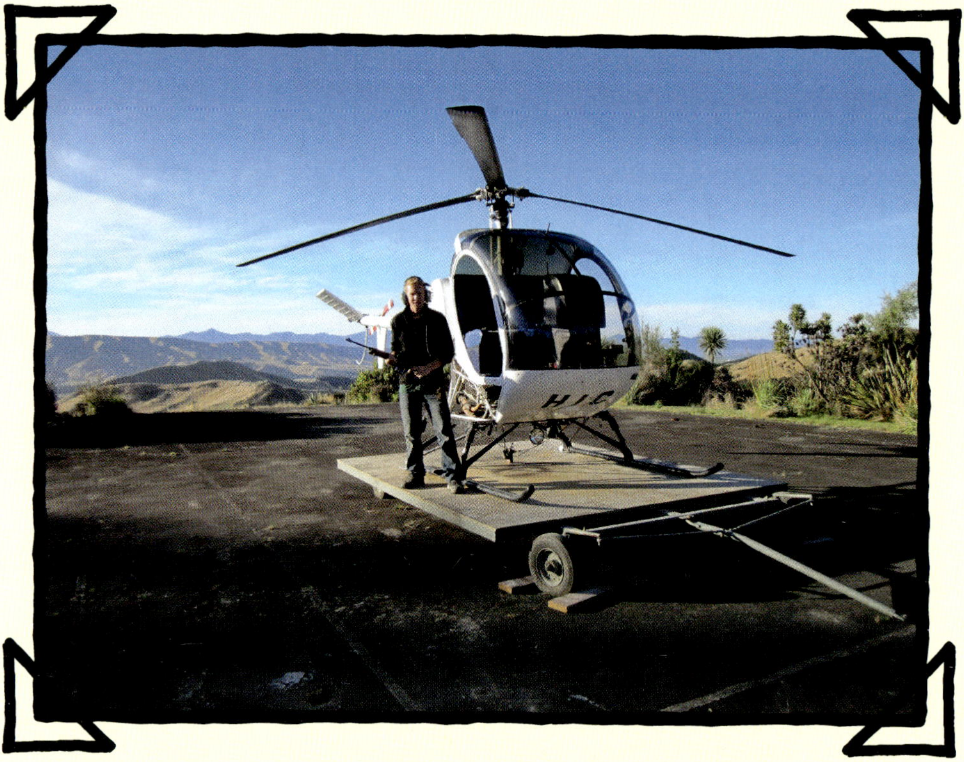

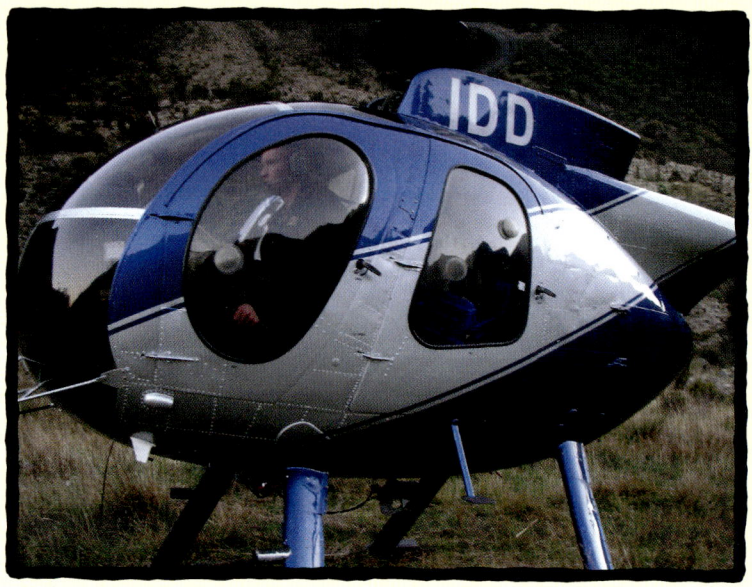

Marc loved shooting deer, whether it was by foot, chopper or truck. Hunting was in his blood.

Marc prepares to take off in his dream-machine Hughes 500D near the big slip in the Irish Burn in Fiordland National Park.

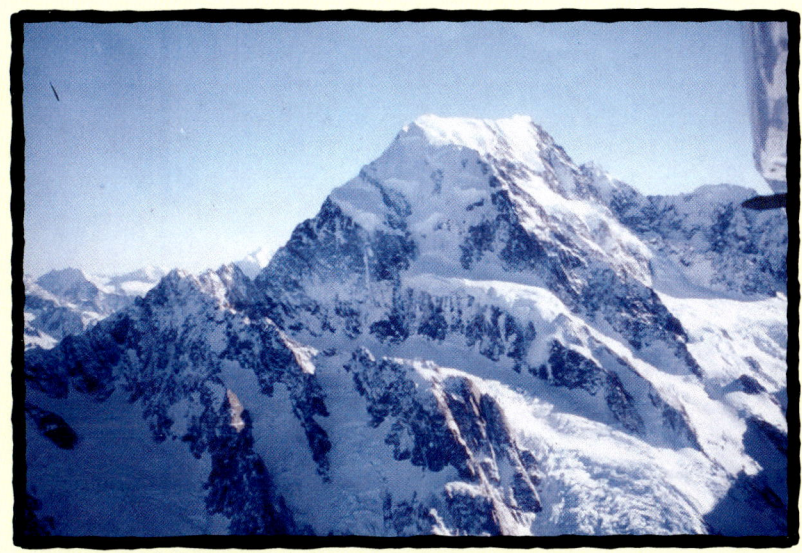

'The Rock'. Whizzing around Aoraki/Mount Cook in my trusty steed, ZK-Really-Jolly-Good.

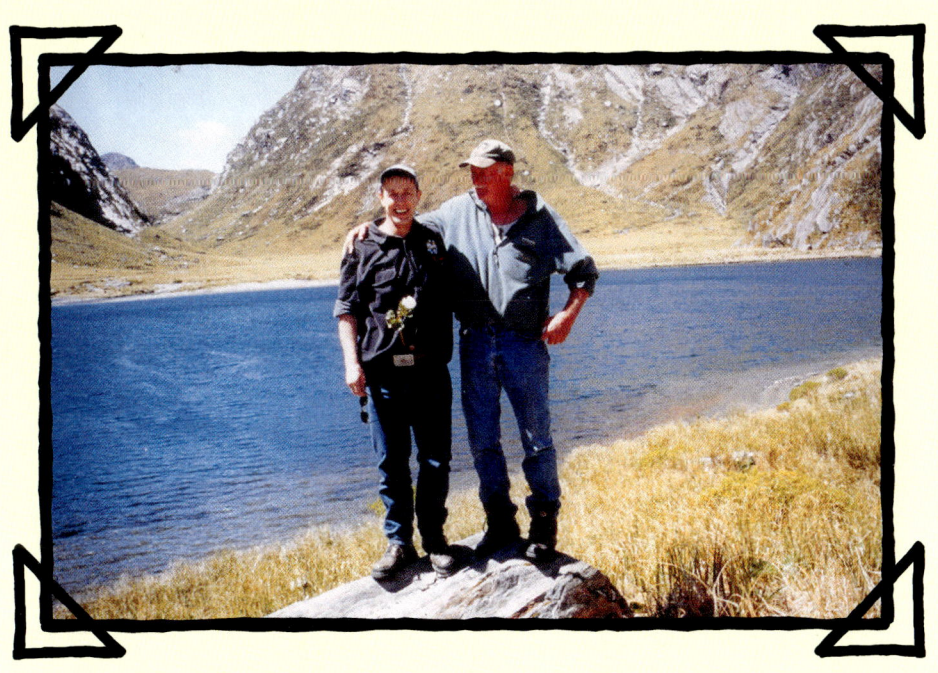

Dave Saxton and me posing at his favourite haunt: the hidden valley near the mighty Okuru River.

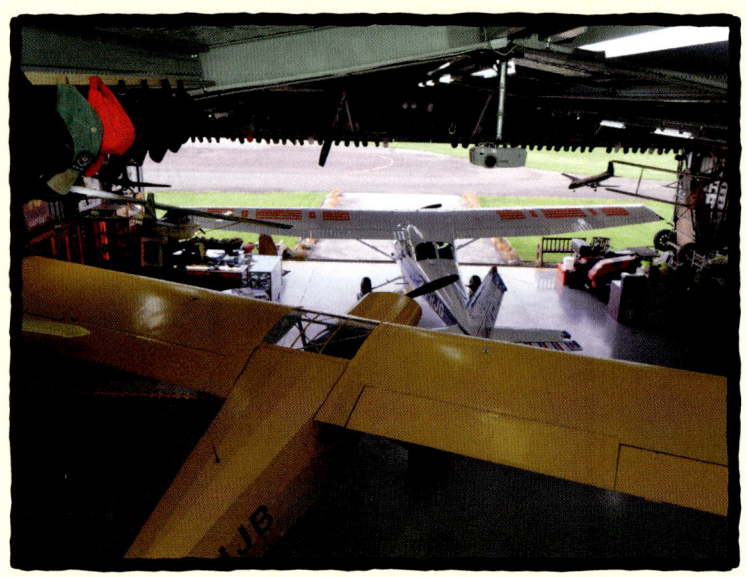

Home sweet home for ZK-Really-Jolly-Good.

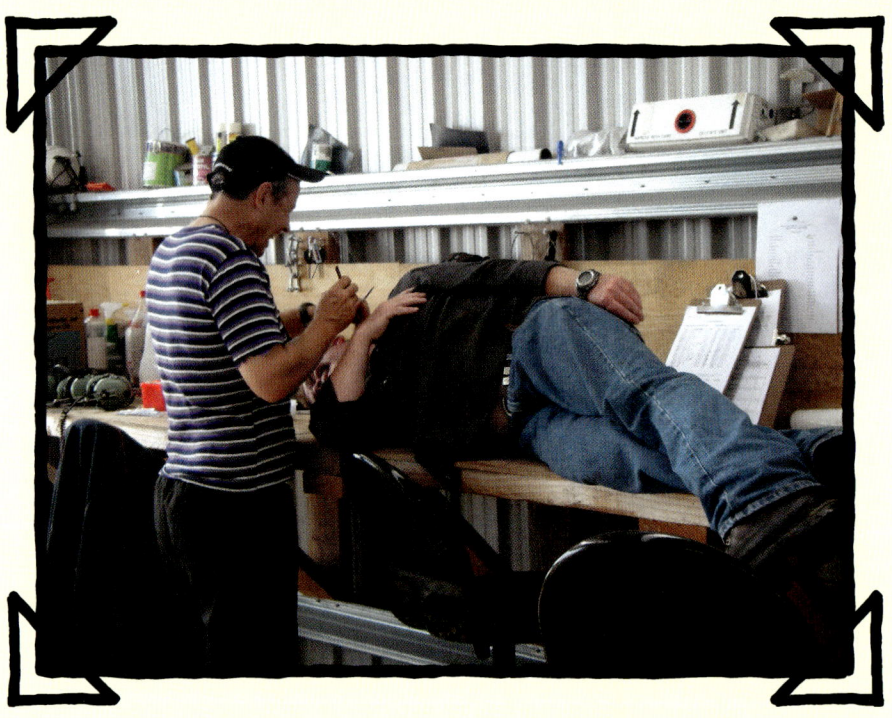

A bit of bush surgery in the back of the hangar adds some variety to the day, and helps out a good Kiwi bloke who wouldn't normally seek out a doctor.

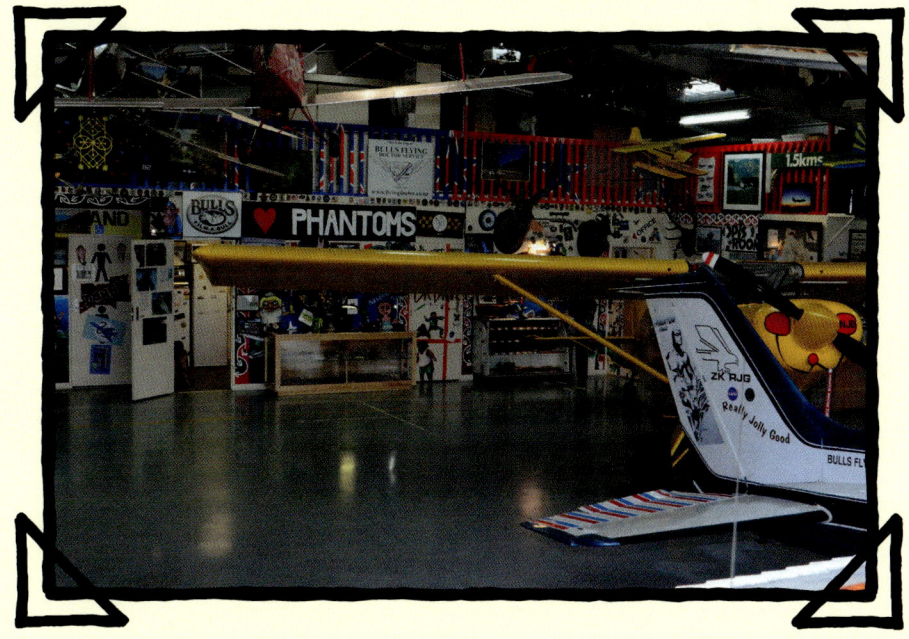

Niki and Anna's awesome artwork abounds at the Marc Baldwin Aerospace Research Centre.

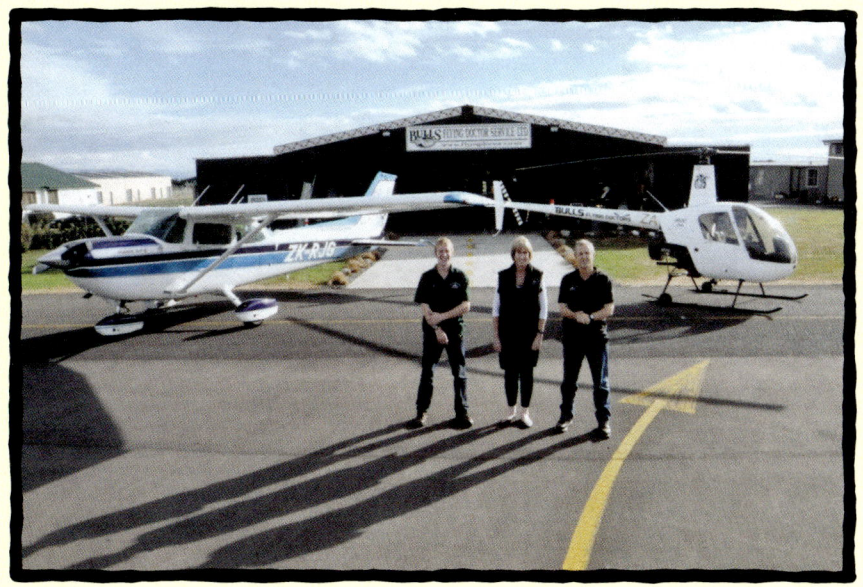

Marc, Rosemary and me at the Bulls Flying Doctor Service aviation medical centre. The place makes me so proud and now has such good memories for me.

A typical mountain river valley located deep within the Southern Alps, no doubt full of big fat deer waiting for us to shoot.

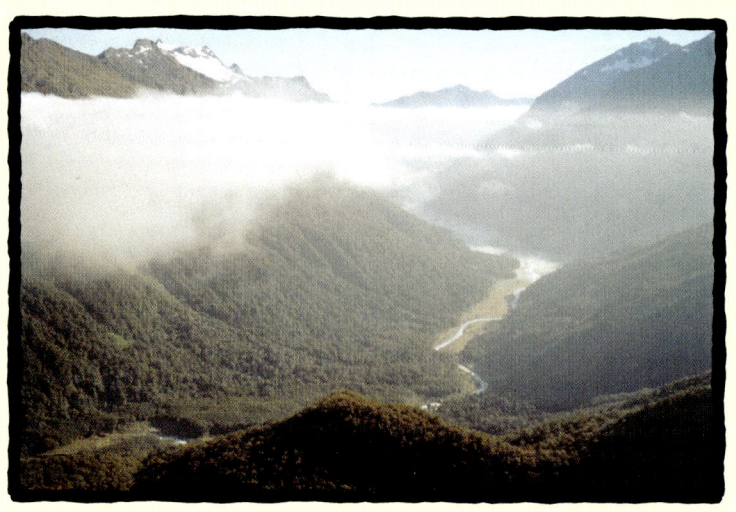

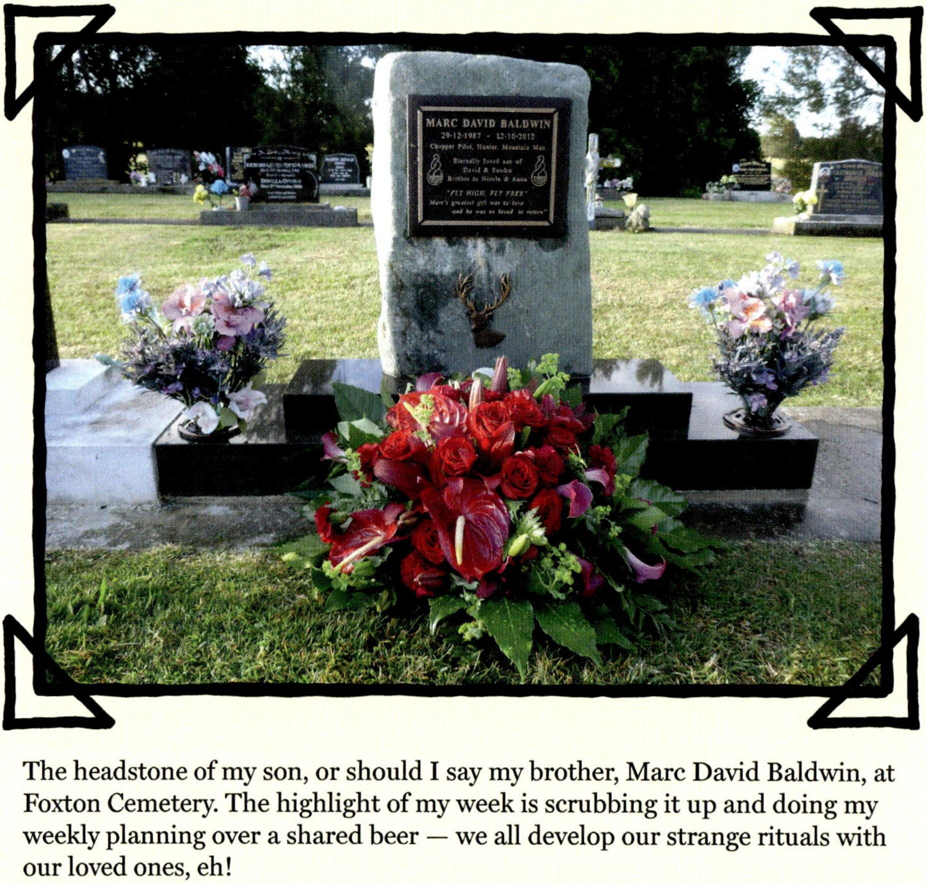

The headstone of my son, or should I say my brother, Marc David Baldwin, at Foxton Cemetery. The highlight of my week is scrubbing it up and doing my weekly planning over a shared beer — we all develop our strange rituals with our loved ones, eh!

always a chance, given I was a deranged loner — and that would spell the end of everything I was trying to build up. The place was full of laughter and good times, all founded on the robust sense of humour we shared. Imagine if some hand-wringing, politically correct dope came in and stuffed everything up!

An example of the good times was when one of our staff members went to the dunny one day, did her business, and somehow managed to get the paper stuck so that when she then wandered off around the practice, the dunny roll spooled out behind her, whirring like a reel when a big fish takes off with a hook in its mouth. I spotted the beginning of this suspicious trail of paper on the ground outside the ladies' and curiously followed it all the way around our practice building corridors, until I ended up at the offender's derrière. There was much rejoicing amongst our little staff and even the red-faced culprit came to see the humorous side to it. I'm sure our patients were quite bemused at the way in which tears would spring to our eyes and we would giggle convulsively, clutching our sore sides for the rest of the day.

In 1999, the Gang of Three flew back into the Landsborough River valley for another hunt. This time we set up at Harper Flat, which has a bush airstrip on it and is a bit further down the valley from the Creswicke Flat Hut. One day, Marc and I were hunting on a ridge above the camp when we heard and then watched a big, shiny Cessna 185 come in to land on the airstrip.

We saw four well-dressed individuals get out of the aeroplane before disappearing into the bush surrounding our camp. But they weren't in there for long. They literally sprinted out of the bush and back to their plane. One of the ladies was in such a hurry that her hat fell off but she just kept on running. The group dived into the aeroplane and immediately took off without doing any sort of preflight inspection that I could see. Marc and I were pissing ourselves laughing; we knew they would have wandered into camp and found a scantily clad Granny Olive busy about her work.

When we returned to camp, we asked Granny Olive if she'd seen anyone while we'd been away.

'Yes, actually,' she replied. 'Some lovely people popped in to say hi. I offered them some scones, but they had to rush. A shame, really, because they seemed very nice.'

Not all of our trips were fun and games, however. In 2000, we flew into Drake Flat on the mighty Waiatoto River to hunt. One evening towards the end of our trip, Marc and I were scouting the banks of the mean, glacial Waiatoto when I spotted a dinghy.

'That'll do the trick for getting across,' I said, pointing it out to Marc.

But when Granny Olive heard about the plan, she was dead against it.

'You'll end up drowning yourselves,' she said.

The next morning, when we reached the riverbank, I told Marc that we would take the dinghy across.

'I don't reckon we should,' he said apprehensively. He had great faith in Granny Olive's judgement. He was probably also thinking, too, about our chamois hunt the year before when he had slipped while we were crossing a snow chute in the Camden Range. It sent us both skating towards the bluffs. Everyone needs reminding every now and again that the mountains don't suffer fools. Sometimes, your first wake-up call is also your last.

'Nah, we'll be right,' I replied.

Marc relented and we crossed the river just fine. We spent the day hunting the steep, beech-clad ridge on the other side, then came back to the river in the late afternoon. The dinghy was there, waiting for us.

It all seemed to happen really fast. I hadn't even got in the boat properly when it skated away from me and flipped, pitching Marc into the swift Waiatoto. His red-blond head disappeared, lost from view in the water made sullen grey and opaque by its burden of rock flour.

'He's gone,' a voice in my head remarked, cool as you like.

I was hanging onto the boat with one hand and my brand-new .270 rifle with the other. I was stuck as long as I stayed like that. There was only one thing to do. I let go of both of them. The boat slipped off downstream, and the rifle faded into the chalky depths of the Waiatoto. I clambered back onto the riverbank and began desperately scanning the water's edge for any sign of my son.

'You fucking idiot. You fucking idiot.'

I don't know whether I was saying it aloud or whether it was in my head. But all of a sudden, I saw him. There was a fallen beech a few metres downstream, and Marc had been swept most of the way underneath it. He had managed to grab a branch and the current was holding him under. His mouth and nose were all that were above the surface, and if he'd relaxed or lost his grip, he would have been a goner.

I rushed to help him out, and then we both sat bawling on the riverbank. It was some time before we were steady enough to get back on our feet and start looking for another way across the river. When we made it back to camp, Granny Olive tore ten thousand strips off me for what I had done. Nothing she said could have made me feel worse. It was a little episode that would haunt my dreams for many years to come.

Once the shock of the near-drowning and the shame and humiliation of my maternal dressing-down had eased a bit, I was able to start to mourn my lovely .270 with its brand-new Weaver scope.

No, I thought. Bugger it, I'm going to try to find it.

As Granny Olive tended to a still-shaking Marc and shot evil glares after me, I returned to the Waiatoto and the scene of our little mishap. I guessed at where I had let the rifle go and tried to calculate how far the current would have carried it before it hit the riverbed. Then I stripped down to my boots and undies, swam out into the middle of the stream and started searching.

It was bitterly cold and you couldn't see your hand in front of your face underwater, so I didn't have long and would have to search by feel. I took a deep breath and ducked under, groping amongst the rocks as the current tugged insistently.

Nothing. I surfaced, a sense of hopelessness beginning to set in. I ducked again, and as I fumbled across the slick stones of the riverbed, my hand bumped and then closed around what was unmistakably a rifle's shoulder strap. I grabbed it with a grip of steel and burst from the water, waving the rifle in triumph. I whooped with delight.

After I'd floundered my way ashore, I couldn't believe my luck when I checked it out and found the scope undamaged without the slightest trace of water inside. All it took was to dry the gun out, and there didn't seem any reason why it would be any the worse for wear.

I made my way back to the hut; although Granny Olive was still raving about how stupid and evil I was, Marc's spirits immediately lifted when he spotted the rifle. He got keen again real quick.

So the very next day, we headed upriver for half an hour and then worked our way up the side of a large slip heading into an area of dense, scrubby leatherwood interspersed with boulders bigger than the size of your average house. I was in front and we were climbing up onto one of these boulders when I came face to face with a chamois sitting right on top. I'm not sure who got the bigger shock. With a high-pitched 'Baaaa!' the chamois took off into the scrub and was gone.

'Aw, man,' Marc moaned.

'Don't give up just yet,' I said. 'Keep your eye on that rock over there. They're inquisitive little buggers. Bet he pops his head up.'

Sure enough, a few minutes later, the chamois popped out of the thick scrub and scaled the rocky outcrop I'd indicated with three nimble bounds. It paused on the top and turned its head towards us. You could almost hear it going: 'Nyah-nyah-nyah-nyah-NYAHH!' at us.

The range was about 350 metres. I marvelled at the clarity of the optics of my nice new Weaver scope, all the clearer for its recent sluicing in the Waiatoto, it seemed, as I nestled the butt of the rifle into my shoulder and settled the cross hairs on a spot just behind the chamois' shoulder. I breathed deeply — in, out, in

— then gently squeezed the trigger. The crack of the rifle rattled around the valley while the chamois gave a spasmodic jerk and tumbled off the rock into the scrub.

'Woohoo!' yelled Marc. 'That fixed old smarty bum!'

Shooting the bloody thing turned out to be the easy part. I got out my compass and took a bearing on the spot.

'I'll make a beeline up there,' I told Marc. 'You stay here. When I'm on my way back, I'll call out. Make sure you yell back or we'll end up getting separated!'

The chamois wasn't dead when I reached it, but it was mortally wounded. I finished it off with my knife, shouldered it and bashed my way back through the nearly impenetrable scrub, following the sound of Marc's voice.

Once we were reunited, we positioned the chamois strategically on a piece of open ground, set up the camera and then squatted by the animal to record the moment for posterity. In the photo, Marc proudly holds the chamois by its little curved horns while I brandish my rifle beside my son and grin like the lucky bastard I was.

This was the first chamois trophy the Gang of Three shot as a team. Granny Olive was over the moon when we got back to the hut, and in no time at all she had an awesome chamois stew simmering in the camp oven.

Ever since I started deerstalking, I have heard every possible argument advanced by hunters around the campfire late at night about what makes for the ultimate rifle and the most reliable telescopic sight for shooting deer. Since that day above the Waiatoto, I have listened to them bang on without ever feeling the need to join in. My Remington .270 and Weaver scope not only survived a beating on the bottom of a glacial river but also shot us a chamois at 350 metres the very next day. I have used nothing else since.

CHAPTER 8

THE BULLS FLYING DOCTOR SERVICE IS BORN

I don't know which of my bush pilot acquaintances first described the traditional aviation medical as 'the gauntlet of fear'. Perhaps it was me . . . God knows I had seen it first-hand often enough.

One of the obligations you have if you hold a pilot's licence is the need to get yourself checked out by a highly trained medical professional every so often to ensure you are sound enough in mind, wind and limb to be trusted with the control of an aircraft. You have to do this every six to twelve months, depending on how old you are, the type of licence you hold and how many people's lives depend on your fitness to fly.

A parade-ground sergeant major would describe the situation for a commercial pilot thus: 'No medical certificate, no flying. No flying means no wages. No wages means you don't eat, and if you don't eat then you don't shit, and if you don't shit you die!'

When I first performed medical exams for pilots in the 1980s, all I did was the actual hands-on examination. I would supply the results to the Civil Aviation Authority (CAA) and they would complete the paperwork and issue the certificate. But in the late 1980s, it was decided that medical practitioners could be trusted to do the paperwork side of things, too. Maybe it was considered more efficient, or maybe the CAA couldn't read doctors' handwriting. Who knows.

Generally speaking, if a pilot wanted to get a CAA Medical Examination prior to the year 2000, he or she would head off to see a Certified CAA Medical Examiner based in a certified location. Certified locations within New Zealand were usually at the pilot's local medical centre.

The trouble with a run-of-the-mill doctor's surgery for a pilot seeking a medical certificate is that they're designed for sick people. Commercial pilots describing their experience of the traditional system indicated an excruciating process with four distinct phases of discomfort.

Phase one began when the pilot walked into a waiting room full of groaning people in various states of distress and decay. With gritted teeth the pilot would push through the huddled masses to the reception desk and hope like hell that the receptionist was in a good mood. If the receptionist was stressed and under pressure — the default state — he or she would be subjected to a lecture delivered at a volume calculated for all in the waiting room to hear. The pilot would then have the paperwork chucked in their direction.

'Sit down,' the receptionist would rasp. 'We'll call you when we can.'

Pairs of sick and rheumy eyes would glare as the pilot guiltily shuffled to a distant corner. The whispering would begin: 'Not sick.' 'Perfectly well.' For the next half-hour, the pilot would try to fill out their CAA medical forms as kids covered in strange rashes screamed and sobbed, old smokers coughed up globules of sputum the size and texture of Bluff oysters, while the receptionist shot the occasional 'Are you still here?' look their way.

Phase two of the gauntlet began when the pilot's name was barked out by the practice nurse. The pilot would slink through the waiting room to the nurse's office. Again, the hope would be that the nurse was in a good mood, because if she (it was usually a she) was under pressure — the default state — the pilot would cop it.

'We're here to treat sick people,' the nurse would mutter. 'What are you doing here, wasting our time with this silly medical?'

Meanwhile, all the basic measurements and tests — height, weight, vision and urine — were performed, with the grumpy old nurse muttering to herself. Of course, if she was experienced in her job, she would have vindictively left blood pressure till last. As she was taking it, she would gasp 'Good God, that's high!' just to get the pilot's blood pressure up a little bit more.

At last the pilot would be delivered to the inner sanctum, the doctor's office itself. The doctor would greet the pilot with a warm and sympathetic smile that would signal phase three of the gauntlet. Naturally enough the doctor would see this appointment with the 'well' pilot as an interesting break from the monotony of a day consulting with moaning, sick people. He or she would bollock on about an uncle who flew Spitfires and virtually won the Battle of Britain single-handed, or the Red Baron in the First World War, of whom the doctor had made a particular, amateur study, or (worst of all) how the doctor was a pilot themself. The pilot would sit there enduring the monologue that he or she had already heard during every other medical they'd ever had. But humouring the doctor was an ace card; it allowed time for blood pressure to settle back. That was almost worth the sore neck from all the nodding.

Eventually, the doctor would become aware of the mutinous rumble from the waiting room and check the time. As the pilot looked on desperately, he or she would swiftly write up notes before laminating the treasured medical certificate and handing it over to the pilot.

Even now, the danger wasn't over. This was phase four, when the pilot must summon every particle of self-control.

'Stay calm. Don't run, you fool.'

The pilot would remember mates who had sustained unnecessary fractures and head injuries from bolting too soon, tripping over sick people in their haste to get away, or even being bowled by a car outside just as they were filling their lungs to utter a gurgling cry of triumph.

After performing one or two medicals for mates, and mates of mates, in the Deep South, it occurred to me that there was no particular need for it to be this way. There was nothing stopping a ruggedly handsome, intrepid and dazzlingly entrepreneurial individual flying into an airstrip and performing aviation medicals in suitably equipped premises nearby. It would be infinitely preferable to calling pilots in to a medical centre. After consulting Sandi, friends and mentors (and floating tea-leaf patterns in a mug of bush tea) that is exactly what I decided to do.

The idea was that I would spend much of my time gadding about the landscape visiting remote localities where assorted characters and legends of the bush and mountain aviation scene would form orderly queues for my services. While I was in these localities, it would be remiss of me not to check out the hunting. And in due course, once he'd finished school and certainly until he was in a position to pursue his own dream, I would involve my usual backcountry sidekick, Marc, in the whole endeavour.

The first step I took towards making the dream a reality was getting a Diploma in Civil Aviation Medicine, the necessary prerequisite for issuing aviation medical certificates. I did the course extramurally through the University of Otago and in double-quick time, too, taking two years to complete instead of the usual three. This was a reflection not only of the guidance of Dr Rob Griffiths, an aviation medicine expert of international standing, but also of how badly I wanted to get my scheme off the ground — as was the fact that I graduated 'with distinction'.

The second and much harder step was upgrading my aeroplane.

Little ZK-Doctor-Never-In was great fun to fly and could even be safely flown through the mountains if the weather was good. It had become part of the family, as all of us, including most of our friends, had had so much fun in it over the years. It had taught me practically everything I knew about flying. However, I accepted it had its limitations, and if I was serious about flying to the deep and mountainous south on a regular basis and in a range of conditions, I needed something better suited to the job. With its 105 HP engine, fixed-pitch propeller and short wings, ZK-Doctor-Never-In just didn't have the performance to get me out of trouble in strong turbulence or downdraughts.

It was with much regret that I eventually sold ZK-Doctor-Never-In. I had already tasked my old buddy Neil Mathieson, the owner of Aero Support at Feilding Aerodrome, with locating a replacement that would meet the needs of my new venture. By sheer luck, he found what seemed to be the perfect aircraft when a Cessna 172 Hawk XP2 turned up for sale. Out of the box, this type of aircraft had the very strong high-lift wings, a powerful 215 HP six-cylinder engine and constant speed unit (CSU) or variable pitch propeller that gave it the performance I needed to fly safely in the mountains. All in all, ZK-Really-Jolly-Good looked the goods, so I persuaded the owner to fly it down to Feilding on 18 September 2000 so we could check it out. Neil examined the airframe and pronounced it 'very good', and he was happy with the engine running times shown in the log. I also noticed that it had a reputable brand of autopilot. Without further ado, I flicked the owner a big fat cheque and ZK-Really-Jolly-Good was mine.

But several things needed attention if ZK-Really-Jolly-Good was to become the flagship plane of what I had come to think of as the Bulls Flying Doctor Service. I'm not shallow, but looks are important and frankly, in its original brown, ZK-Really-Jolly-Good looked like a flying turd. I engaged the services of legendary local painter, Ron Wood. I wanted blue and white, while Granny Olive wanted purple. So blue, white and purple it was, and every time I do a preflight check or I polish her up (which I do every 50 to 100 flying hours), I still admire Ron's handiwork.

I went even further. If I was to be a flying doctor, I also wanted the world to know. When I pass overhead, all those eyes flung to the heavens watching me go can read 'Flying Doctor' under my wings. And as for anyone looking down from above — you know who you are — I can be identified by bold red strips on the topside of my wings and tailplane. This isn't so much to send messages to the alien mothership, as those with paranormal inclinations have suggested: it's more to do with the fact that currently there are six aircraft missing without trace south of Haast. If I were to go down in the bush or the mountains, those bold splashes of colour just might be the difference between me being found or me becoming number seven. If I crashed, I wanted to be found as soon as possible, not spend my last days immobilised and starving to death while listening to search aircraft flying overhead unable to see me and ZK-Really-Jolly-Good hidden under the bush canopy.

The new aircraft meant that the 'Skunk Works' (the name we had bestowed on our hangar at RNZAF Base Ohakea) would need modification, too, to accommodate the greater wingspan. So I roped in my cuzzy-bro Richard Speedy to do the honours, as surreptitiously as we could, because while I still had a good relationship with the base, I preferred not to draw any more attention to myself than was strictly necessary.

THE FLYING DOCTOR

A lot of the airports where I proposed to do pilot medicals were very remote and a long way from Bulls. To get a good head start on the day's flight schedule, it would be necessary to take off very early in the morning when it was dark and often cloudy. I decided to transplant the instrument flight rules (IFR) avionics from ZK-Doctor-Never-In to ZK-Really-Jolly-Good, and added a few extra gadgets — a back-up electric artificial horizon, a visual flight rules (VFR) GPS and a high-frequency (HF) radio — to make my IFR flying safer. The HF radio allows me to call up the Maritime Operations Centre at Avalon in Lower Hutt using the VHF radio channel 16; this is very useful when I am tripping around out to sea off Fiordland. Praise the lord for technology!

On the other hand, too much technology can make you lazy and complacent. I tried out a couple of the collision avoidance systems available on the market, but I found they often gave misleading (and dodgy) information. At one time, I was happily flying along at 10,000 feet and the collision avoidance system burst into life: 'Emergency! Aircraft same altitude!! Pull up!!!' It scared the living shit out of me, and I called up Air Traffic Control to see who I was about to hit. They assured me there was nothing in my vicinity.

Even worse were the times I was flying along and other aircraft zipped past with the wretched collision avoidance system staying serenely quiet. I did the only decent thing: I took it out and used it for target practice. Since then, I have concentrated on keeping my own lookout for other aircraft and closely monitoring the radio for situation reports from other aircraft.

THE BULLS FLYING DOCTOR SERVICE IS BORN

One trick I have learned in my time as a doctor is that it's useful being your aviation techo's GP, especially if you know they have a phobia for hypodermic needles. The needle-phobic Neil and the boys at Aero Support have done a great job keeping ZK-Really-Jolly-Good's engine going and, in the best tradition of dressing mutton up as lamb, have also added a few modern sensors to ensure greater efficiency and safe running. These included GAMI fuel injectors with an EDM-700 Engine Analyser and digital flow gauge to allow more accurate leaning of fuel at altitude (meaning the adjustment of the proportion of fuel added to the fuel–air mixture as the air thins and oxygen becomes more scarce) and more accurate and rapid troubleshooting if anything should go wrong. I also got a sump pad warmer installed to preheat the oil before take-off and I am sure this feature, along with good in-flight engine management, has been a major factor in keeping the engine going. The type of engine powering ZK-Really-Jolly-Good is expected to require a full overhaul by the time it has done 2000 hours. At the time of writing, the engine has done 3500 hours without missing a beat. (Doctor touches wood.)

As a breed, the Cessna 172 airframe has a proven safety record, but I thought I would add a few bits and bobs to enhance it further still, such as flap flow strips and vortex generators, which are little vanes and fins that improve the aerodynamics and give greater lift and performance. I also installed a proper parachute door on the co-pilot's side. This not only provided reassurance that all I have to do to escape the aircraft in the event of an in-flight emergency is to scramble over my shrieking passenger and fling open the door, but it also helps when loading medical equipment in and out of the aircraft. And while the door has a metal frame, it's mostly clear Perspex so it also greatly improves my visibility. Most of the time I fly alone with the co-pilot's seat taken out; on long flights I can set the autopilot and work away on my laptop with the most magnificent views imaginable from my office window.

The back seats have been replaced with a large wooden cabinet built by local joinery genius Cameron Stohers, in which I can efficiently stow all of my medical equipment, emergency gear, spare parts for the aircraft, and IFR flight manuals. As for the medical gear I take around the country with me, it is high quality, very portable and fits compactly into two packs that are strapped tightly into the back of the aircraft in case of severe turbulence. Over the years I have found that it's important to have back-up gear like a spare ECG or audiogram — fancy instruments for imaging the heart and measuring hearing respectively — which are stowed away separately.

If you are a nervous flyer (the sort of person who dutifully stares at the flight attendant as they do that silly mime with the life jacket) spare a thought for your pilot. Pilots know far more about what might go wrong than you do and, if they're good pilots, they're constantly thinking about disaster because the best way to be prepared is to rehearse in your mind what you will do in the unlikely event of an emergency.

I have always been a good boy scout (dib dib dob dob!) and like to be prepared. That has meant getting the best advice and equipment from people like Tony Rolleston at Marinair. The most likely emergency that could happen to ZK-Really-Jolly-Good is an in-flight engine failure. If it happens at night over land, or during the day while flying over cloud-covered mountainous terrain, then I would do the decent thing and bail out using my large red-and-white-canopied parachute. On the other hand, if the engine failed over water, I have an inflatable dinghy at the ready, along with a pair of goggles and a really good survival jacket with a small compressed air cylinder attached to it that would deliver enough air for five minutes' normal breathing. Such is the nature of the Cessna 172 that if I did ditch, the plane would sink by the nose pretty much immediately. But I am confident that with the goggles and the air bottle, I'd not only have enough time to get out of the cockpit, but also to grab a few crays while I was down there.

I had Brian Carter, an upholsterer in Bulls, work his magic on my survival vest, adding various little pockets, Velcro and clips, which all make the oxygen cylinder, whistle and flashlight accessible and comfortable to wear. In part, of course, I'm trusting Murphy's law that the harder I prepare for something, the less likely it is to happen. (Doctor crosses fingers.)

When I started flying around Aoraki/Mount Cook and over the Tasman Glacier, I would keep an eye out for places to land if the engine failed — most pilots subconsciously do this as they trip around the countryside. Most of the Tasman Valley is strewn with massive boulders, making a forced landing without power very risky, so the only likely spot seemed to be the tranquil Tasman Terminal Lake. This was all good and dandy in my mind until one day, when Sandi and I went for a guided boat trip on the lake. The guide asked everyone who was in the boat to put their hand in the freezing water for more than ten seconds. I dipped my hand in without hesitation but the water was so cold that I developed severe pain and cramp well before the 10 seconds were up. This little lesson made me rethink my ditching plans in this part of the country, and really got me deliberating about the dangers of cold water.

This issue of ditching into cold water and developing hypothermia has occupied my mind ever since I started flying. In the early days of flying over Cook Strait I had tried using a full ex-RNZAF immersion suit. But it took almost 15 minutes to put it on, and just as long to take it off at my destination; it was also desperately hot and uncomfortable to wear en route, to say nothing of the fact that it made me look like a prize dick. I still have it, but because of its impracticality and the fact it is the aviation fashion equivalent of flared trousers, it is now a museum piece.

Two other essential pieces of emergency gear I purchased for ZK-Really-Jolly-Good since starting out are a satellite phone and a satellite tracking system. The satellite phone is ideal for calling up the emergency services from the ground in even the most isolated mountain valleys. In the meantime, the satellite tracking system built into the plane fires a signal every two minutes via the Iridium network — a global version of your everyday, national cellphone network — to some satellite high in the sky, giving precise information about my airspeed, altitude and position which can be remotely recorded. It's an amazing system and was installed by Chris Hinch of TracPlus and John Wyllie of Flightcell. I find it very reassuring that someone will know where I am if I end up wandering off on a sightseeing detour up some hidden mountain valley — as I often do — and crash.

Once my new aircraft was set up, I knew I could finally let ZK-Doctor-Never-In go. What made it all twice as hard was the fact that the new owner taxied my old aircraft into a ditch a couple of months later, damaging it beyond repair. I have a rule of never criticising other pilots for mishaps, because there but for the grace of God, and so on, but I made an exception in his case. But of course, not long after deploring what happened to poor old ZK-Doctor-Never-In, I was taxiing a mate's beautiful Cessna 182 on a farm airstrip when I got distracted by something going on in the cockpit. I looked up just in time to see the edge of a big, flooded pothole looming. It was too late to do anything about it and, as Fred Dagg once put it, 'Over she goes!' I nosed right into the muck and did much costly damage to the engine and propeller. Talk about eating humble pie!

=

By the beginning of 2001, just as my new venture was about ready to take off, the good old government looked like it was going to clip my wings. The Civil Aviation Amendment Bill (No. 2) was introduced, which would have reinstated the stupid centralised system of medical certification, so that the only input a doctor could have would be to report the findings of a medical exam. There was no money in flying to, say, Te Anau and poking and prodding a few pilots if I couldn't charge them for the whole service, including issuing the certificate. I was so hot under the collar about this particular measure that I presented myself to Parliament on 7 March 2001 and made submissions to the select committee considering the bill. The centralisation provision had disappeared by the time the bill became law the following year, so it's hard to resist the conclusion that it was my impassioned oratory that moved the lawmakers. Well, mine and the several hundred others from the aviation industry and the Aviation Medical Society who also opposed the bill.

After this narrowly avoided catastrophe, and by the time the Civil Aviation Authority had bestowed the honour of being an accredited aviation medical inspector upon David Edward Baldwin — or AMA1 number 1043 as the tattoo in my left armpit has it — there was nothing stopping my dream of flying. I enlisted the help of the accountant who did the books for the Bulls Medical Centre Ltd, Hugh Glendinning, to assist me in setting up the Bulls Flying Doctor Service as a limited liability company. I didn't know where I stood in terms of intellectual property with the name: the Australians seemed to have a bit of an interest in the general concept of flying doctors, so to head off any legal unpleasantness I got a signwriter on the job to make me up a sign to display at the Bulls Medical Centre:

Home of the Bulls Flying Doctor Service

and our subsidiary organisation

The Australian Flying Doctor Service

That should clear it up, I thought. But funnily enough you can always tell the Australian visitors to Bulls by the huffing and puffing they do over that sign. Perhaps it's because I left the 'Royal' off the name of the Aussie outfit. That was quite deliberate. I know it's been a while coming, but I remain confident that we'll be given the right to call ourselves the Royal Bulls Flying Doctor Service any day now. Then we'll happily give the Aussies their royal due, too. In the meantime, we call ourselves the Not-So-Royal Bulls Flying Doctor Service, or NSRBFDS for short.

=

Enough of the backroom corporate stuff! The whole point of the NSRBFDS was to do some actual flying, so the next important task for me was establishing satellite facilities that we would need to ply our trade. The first of these — fittingly, given it was there where the whole concept was born — was at Haast in South Westland. The township of Haast is located on the southern side of the huge Haast River on a thin strip of swampy coastal plain that separates the massive mountain chain of the Southern Alps from the wild Tasman Sea. It's an absolutely awesome place to fly in to from any direction.

What was to become known as the Haast Aerospace Research Centre was set up in the base of Heliventures, the tourism venture belonging to the Saxton family and located on their farm. It was only a kilometre or so away from the Haast airstrip, but I didn't have to worry about getting myself and my gear from the strip to the clinic, because Dave or Morgie would always be there with a chopper, ready to go. At the time, Dave, Debbie, Morgan and Lisa Saxton were doing a roaring trade. The whole place rocked with the sound of whining turbine engines starting up and the wocka-wocka of rotor blades bending under the stress of rapid take-offs or landings. There was a constant flow of hunters, tourists, odd-bod hermits and pilots coming in and out of the place, which made it all very exciting and quite the place to be.

The NSRBFDS clinic room was unique as a surgery in the early days because it came complete with a cage at the front door containing a large white parrot which often squawked 'Fuck off' as I passed it by. I don't know why, as I was always quite civil. Nor am I sure what happened to the parrot in the end, but word was the abuse it dished out eventually tipped someone over the edge and it got taken out the back and shot. Knowing West Coasters like I do, I find that easy to believe. A terrible, terrible business. God, I loved that parrot. NOT!

I took care to equip the clinic with ancient medical gear and a variety of even older medical antiques that everyone had a lot of fun with. When I wasn't there Dave Saxton or Morgan would often nip into the clinic room, grab something like an old stethoscope and then chase visitors around the farm trying to record their blood pressure or hear the sounds of their heart. Sometimes Dave would raid my store cupboard and sidle up to visitors with a fistful of condoms or, when he really wanted to be creepy, the offer of a sneaky enema. So far as I know, no one ever took him up on it. Morgan, after a few beers, dressed up in the Skyhawk pilot's zoom bag — the technical name for a fighter pilot's onesie — that I had given him and arranged a photo shoot, much to the amusement of all concerned.

Given how far south Haast is, it occurred to me it would be handy to have bases en route. I already had contacts at Hokitika (Hoki). In February 2001, I met up with a couple of old-hand West Coast aviation enthusiasts, Murray Bowes and Jim Jamieson, who, along with Rob Daniels, helped me organise the use of a room under the old control tower at the airport where I could do pilot medical examinations. With the room sorted, the Hoki Aerospace Research Centre was born and has since become a very important hub for the NSRBFDS for a number of reasons.

Firstly, Hokitika Airport has an IFR approach, so I can land or take off in the dark or in bad weather. This meant I could land at Hoki very early in the morning under IFR, potter around the Coast doing my aviation medicals using visual flight rules (VFR) during daylight hours, and then be back at Hoki Airport just before dark. I can refuel the aircraft, get my gear repacked and fill up my thermos with coffee, safe in the knowledge that I can do a full IFR departure in the dark. It certainly takes the pressure off.

Secondly, we have been blessed at Hoki with a succession of airport managers. Nothing has ever seemed to be a problem — whether it be getting the lights turned on for an unscheduled take-off or parking the aircraft for an overnighter in a secure place with good lighting.

Thirdly, with over 30 years' experience studying and predicting the often wildly changeable West Coast weather, Mark Crompton, the local meteorologist, has saved my butt more than a few times. Luckily he has a soft spot for quality wine, so we have developed a reciprocal contra relationship, which we refer to as the 'weather-for-wine' arrangement.

And, finally, Joe Beckett's De Havilland Café at the airport is a great place to have a good bullshit session with some of the mates I have developed over the years — and coming from Bulls I know I am very well qualified to run a bullshit session. Bruce Watson is one such mate; he owns the bookshop in Hoki and shares my interest in the outdoors and the history of the West Coast, especially pioneer explorers like Charlie 'Mr Explorer Douglas' (1840–1916) and William 'Arawata Bill' O'Leary (1865–1947). Bruce always keeps me posted if any new or old books come out about these tough old-timers. Then there's also good old Bevan Climo, a master greenstone (pounamu) carver, whose knowledge of the Coast is immense. He often pops up for a cuppa when I am passing through. Bevan has a deep understanding of Maoridom, especially the spiritual side of things, for which I have developed a bit of a bent myself. Apart from that he keeps me well stocked with pounamu shepherd's whistles that I gift to my special mates around the country.

—

Soon after setting up the Hokitika Aerospace Research Centre, I headed south to Fox Glacier airstrip with the aim of setting up a small clinic down there. Fox Glacier looks like the kind of place that Peter Jackson would have had to invent if he'd wanted to set *The Lord of the Rings* in unbelievable scenery. It's so pretty it's idiotic, sitting there under the morning shadow of Aoraki/ Mount Cook. I had to be there! After all, my family has history with old Cloud Piercer: Granny Olive almost got to the top several times, and was only a matter of metres from the top on her closest attempt when she got caught in a rock fall and had to be carted off to horsepital.

To find suitable premises, I enlisted the help of James and Debbie Scott. James is one of the many Scotts descended from Andrew Scott, who settled here over a hundred years ago. James not only runs a large farm in the Karangarua River flats, but also has a very successful heli-tourism operation. His passion lies in the mountains and hunting — very few people know South Westland better than James. Together with John Sullivan — another descendant of local pioneering stock — we found what seemed like a suitable room at the Fox Glacier Fire Station. After it proved to be a hassle lugging my medical gear from the airport to the station, I learned that the Skydive Fox Glacier boys working on the airstrip had a spare room. It was perfect, and it initiated a long friendship with an awesome group of guys that included Rod 'Sarge' Miller, John Kerr, Chris MacDonald, Greg Rowan, Rod Davis and many others. I found the skydivers to be more or less kindred spirits, taking issue with them only over the wisdom of jumping out of a perfectly serviceable aeroplane. Even on this, my attitude softened as the years went by, and eventually, in 2009, I did something I swore I would never do. Yep, against my better judgement, I did a tandem skydive jump with the Sarge, and I have to say that falling out of an aeroplane at 12,000 feet near Aoraki/Mount Cook was a thrill that can't be described in mere words. You just have to do it.

CHAPTER 9

BECOMING RESPECTABLE

It was yet another glorious day in the most beautiful place in the world: Haast. Morgan Saxton met me at the airstrip and whisked me to the Haast Aerospace Research Centre by the farmhouse. On the way, he told me he had a real treat in store for me.

Oh, goodie, I thought. Chamois. Maybe even Himalayan tahr.

'Geoff and I are gunna take you fishing!' Morgie told me.

My disappointment must have been written all over my face. I had no complaints about the company: I couldn't think of any blokes, besides Marc, with whom I'd rather spend time than Morgie and Geoff Robson. Geoff was a very old friend of Morgie and Dave's who ran a fishing operation with his two sons, Mike and Spud, at Neils Beach just down the road. Geoff and Morgie often hung out together, and often got up to mischief. The trouble I had was *fishing*.

'It'll be great,' Morgie reassured me. 'Just you wait.'

I worked my way through my list of medicals. Just before I was scheduled to finish, I heard the unmistakable whine of a Hughes 500D turbine starting up on the pad outside the clinic. I'd sort of hoped Morgie would have reconsidered the fishing expedition in the meantime, but no. As soon as I emerged, blinking, into the sunshine, he was there to grab me.

'Fishing!' He clapped his hands.

I fear I may have been a touch surly as I climbed into the chopper with Geoff and Morgie. We lifted off and swung out over the beach and out to sea. This struck me as a bit odd, because the local trout were normally to be found in the big rivers that lay in the exact opposite direction. Morgie made no move to turn around and if Geoff thought there was something odd about the fact that the next trout stream in this direction would be in Tasmania, he wasn't giving anything away. The sun, low over the horizon dead ahead, glittered impassively on his shades.

I began to suspect this was no ordinary fishing trip.

Fifteen miles out to sea, a boat appeared ahead of us. It was a commercial fishing vessel and it was hove to. A lone figure stood with his feet planted on the gently rocking deck, hands on hips, watching us come in. I knew that boat. It was Spud Robson down there.

Morgie brought the chopper to a hover over the boat while Geoff got a fishing line ready. He opened a door and lowered an empty hook. Spud stood motionless as the wash from the rotors whipped the sea around the boat to froth. Then he reached into a large plastic bin on the deck alongside him and hooked a huge fish onto the line.

'Got one!' exclaimed Geoff, and reeled in a giant bluenose.

We repeated the exercise eight or nine more times.

'This is fishing!' whooped Geoff, and I had to agree. Then, with a jaunty wave to Spud, Morgie wheeled the chopper around and we swept back towards the coast. We landed right next to ZK-Really-Jolly-Good. I loaded my medical gear, a full flask of coffee and 10 huge bluenose into the aircraft, waved goodbye to Geoff and Morgie and took off on the three-and-a-half-hour trip back to Ohakea.

Once on the ground, I now faced the unusual problem of how to deal with all that fish. Our freezer was pretty small, and there was no way I was going to let all that beautiful, fresh bluenose go to waste . . . Thus began 'The Great Bluenose Giveaway Tour'.

Happy, then, were the folk I spotted on my trip home: a cleaner, a semi-drunken airman weaving his way homeward, two security guards patrolling the perimeter, the gate guard, a friendly policeman parked by the road to Bulls, the petrol station attendant and then a couple of our friends. Each received a bloody great fish, courtesy of the Not-So-Royal Bulls Flying Doctor Service. I was left with a single fish, and it was so big I could hardly fit the bloody thing into our freezer.

=

By now, I was doing aviation medicals all over the show, and Marc and I had embarked on the process of setting up the infrastructure

— a bunch of satellite clinics — in suitable localities nationwide. I'll admit our selection process incorporated a strong bias towards the rugged, picturesque and deer-infested parts of the country.

The feedback I received from my clients was rapturous, and the rate at which new enquiries were coming in indicated word of mouth was working well. But there was some negativity. A few incumbent aviation medical doctors working in or near the various localities I was visiting phoned me to complain that I was encroaching on their turf. Some used language that would have made an aged barmaid from the East End of London blush! I was quite unfazed by that because, as I pointed out to them, if they were providing the kind of service that my clients wanted, there would be no work for me.

It also filtered back to me that some pilots were openly sceptical about the quality of my work, and there were apparently dark mutterings around, to the effect that I was doing aviation medicals out of the boot of a car.

To try to change this perception, I delivered a talk to the Aviation Medical Society of New Zealand conference in late 2001. I gather some of those present were among the sadly misguided individuals who had been muttering about me, but when they saw that my presentation was generally well-received — most aviation doctors just love to fly, and the emotion I read in the majority of the faces in the audience before me was raw, naked envy — they kept quiet. There arose a broad recognition that 'a man's gotta do what a man's gotta do', and resistance, which had always been useless, began to fade away.

It certainly helped my case that officialdom smiled upon my venture. You're fighting an uphill battle if, on top of everything else a new business faces, you've got the feds on your case. Once I had decided that I was going to do aviation medicals away from my home territory, I took the precaution of keeping the Civil Aviation Authority's Central Medical Unit (CMU) informed of what we were doing. The doctors at CMU were very supportive, not only because they could see the value in it, but also because certain changes in the way the certification process happened had made the paperwork more onerous for already overworked rural doctors, and many had given it away. It was therefore most convenient for the CMU that I was there to step into the breach. Anyway, I was very thankful for the support from Dougal Watson, Claude Preitner, Mike Drane and Pooshan Navathe.

All the same, and while I was still visiting the letterbox daily in the hope of finding my Royal Charter amongst the mail, I thought it would be prudent to seek legitimacy for what I was doing in whatever form I could. Brandishing a particularly large hypodermic syringe, I suggested to Neil Mathieson that if he felt inclined to nominate me for an Aviation Safety Award, I might be able to find other ways of administering his medicine. Boy, he must really be scared of needles! Not only did he nominate me, but the amount of support he was able to drum up in the aviation community saw me duly awarded the 2003 award. As expected, the crowds went wild, the police were called to quell the ensuing riot and I was inundated with sponsorship money and support — and then I woke up. But nearly as good, I no longer heard any of that negative gossip.

Both *New Zealand Doctor* magazine and the CAA's *Vector* magazine gave me very favourable write-ups. In its 'Know your medical examiner' column, *Vector* referred to me as 'the energetic

Dr Dave Baldwin' and thoroughly approved of the concept of the NSRBFDS offering pilot-friendly aviation medical services.

Dougal Watson, the CMU's Principal Medical Officer, even tagged along on one of my forays to Motueka and Blenheim. This proved very handy, because a couple of the pilots whom I was examining had issues that would need escalation to the CMU to sort out. You can imagine how impressed my clients were when I produced the Principal Medical Officer himself on the spot!

In April 2001, I made my first visit on official NSRBFDS business to Aoraki/Mount Cook. It made sense to establish a base there, as I had a cousin, Malcolm Walls, who lived with his wife Roseanne just down the road at Twizel. Plus the region is just amazing. It's big country with a little township nestled right at the feet of the tallest mountains in the country, making aviation bloody dodgy and bloody awesome all at once.

Once I was on the ground, Malcolm met me and introduced me to Wayne McMillan, chief pilot for Mount Cook Ski Planes which had been founded in the 1950s by Harry Wigley. Wigley had invented the concept of retractable skis for landing on glaciers and snowfields. That probably took some gonads back in 1955 when he first tried it out; and the people who fly for Mount Cook Ski Planes these days remain true to that type. Spending all their time in this place, they're just about the only people on earth I have ever really had occasion to envy.

Wayne and Malcolm had arranged space for me in the

Department of Conservation and New Zealand Land Search and Rescue (LandSAR) first-aid room. This turned out to be too far from the airfield to be practical, given the gear I have to lug from the plane to the examination room. Ah, well, it's always the thought that counts.

On reflection, they realised there was a little room upstairs in the Mount Cook Terminal Building that I could use, and so the Mount Cook Aerospace Research Unit was born. The Terminal Building is new and flash; the only thing to be regretted is that it replaces the old terminal, which burned down on Friday, 30 June 2000, taking with it any amount of priceless memorabilia of Harry Wigley and other pioneers of the Mount Cook operation.

Mount Cook has become a favourite destination for me. Back then, half of the appeal was spending time with Malcolm and Roseanne, who had an airstrip on their high-country farm. I would stay with them, and Malcolm and I would sit up late discussing local history and talking over the business of flying in the hills. Malcolm was a guru on both and I loved listening to his theories on some of the aviation mysteries from that part of the world. Where, we wondered, was the Cessna 172 belonging to the Turner family, which disappeared with Roy Turner, his wife and two young kids en route from Tekapo to Fox Glacier in the winter of 1983? And where was the DH.90 Dragonfly flown by Brian Chadwick, missing with the pilot and four passengers (two of them on their honeymoon) on a scenic flight from Christchurch to Milford Sound in February 1962?

The ski-plane pilots, with their wide knowledge of flying in and around those huge mountains in the Aoraki/Mount Cook National Park, were very helpful in filling in the gaps in my mountain flying experience. Once, early on in the piece, I finished doing a few aviation medicals at the Mount Cook Aerospace Research Unit and was preparing to fly to my next stop at Fox Glacier. The distance is only 16 nautical miles but involves a climb to over 7500 feet to get through even the lowest pass to Fox Glacier. On this particular day, there was a 50-knot southwesterly wind at 10,000 feet, which came with a severe turbulence warning for the region. When I looked out the window of the Mount Cook Terminal Building, I could see a big stack of lenticular clouds building up over the peaks of Aoraki/Mount Cook, a sure sign of high winds. It wasn't looking good for getting to Fox Glacier, but just before ringing the pilots I had lined up over there to postpone their medicals, I asked Wayne and Ross Anderson, who were the duty pilots at Mount Cook on the day, if they thought I could get over the Alps safely in the conditions.

'No sweat,' they said. 'Just track up the eastern side of the Tasman Glacier and when you're abeam Malte Brun, turn left and shoot through the Graham Saddle. You won't feel a bump.'

Either this was great advice or humour of the blackest kind. I looked deep into their eyes to ensure they weren't setting me up for a hiding. They passed 'The Dr Dave Patent Bullshit Detection and Mind-Reading Test', so I decided to give it a go. I did an extra-long goodbye to everyone in case I didn't make it and wandered out on the tarmac to ZK-Really-Jolly-Good. I could just about hear the 'Last Post' as I loaded my gear and preflighted the aircraft. I tied all my gear down extra tight just in case I did end up in severe turbulence.

From the moment I took off, it didn't look too good; it was already a bit bumpy from low-level turbulence. But once I started climbing through the call-up (or visual reporting) points of Rotten Tommy and Murchison Corner on the eastern side of the Tasman Valley, it all smoothed out. The amazing spectacle of the ruffled and jumbled Tasman Glacier, slumped in its basin of grim, grey stone, unrolled below me as I aimed for the tall, shapely and snow-capped Minarets. As I passed 8000 feet, I looked left to the massive presence of Aoraki/Mount Cook, now proudly sporting seven or eight layers of smooth lenticular clouds like a stack of Chinese coolie hats. How I managed to keep a firm grip on the control column with my palms sweating like that, I'll never know. I clenched my teeth and braced for the hammering I was surely about to endure.

At 9000 feet I levelled off. After reaching Malte Brun and nodding respectfully at the 10,495-foot peak that Mum climbed in the 1970s, I turned west towards the Graham Saddle, named after Peter and Alec Graham, a couple of great mountaineers of the early 1900s who pioneered it as a crossing of the Southern Alps. I edged ZK-Really-Jolly-Good towards the low point in the snowy rampart and then slid on through it. I was finally on the West Coast, and I'd got there without a single bump!

'Thanks, boys!' I yelled, looking left and down towards the Mount Cook Terminal Building which I could still see way down below me to the southeast.

That's why local knowledge is so important when mountain flying; the harsh reality is that most of the high ridges and major saddles of the Southern Alps are still lightly dusted with bits of aircraft debris from previous accidents that happened when pilots failed to stick to the basics of mountain flying or neglected to seek advice from local aviators.

From the Graham Saddle, I descended and landed at Fox Glacier airstrip, where it was blowing a fair gale. As I began unloading my medical gear from the plane, a pilot mooched over.

'Where you come from?' he asked.

'Mount Cook,' I replied nonchalantly.

His eyebrows shot up.

'How the hell did you get over from there in this wind?'

'No sweat,' I drawled. 'In a southwesterly wind, just whizz up the eastern side of the Tasman Valley and come through the Graham Saddle. Easy, yeah, real easy. I do it all the time . . .'

I think I spoiled the effect by blushing and failing to meet his eye.

—

Over the first two years or so of our operation, Marc and I set up 11 other 'aerospace research centres' besides Palmy and Hoki: four others in the North Island (Gisborne, Hastings, Masterton and Taupo) and seven others in the South Island (Blenheim, Motueka, Omarama, Mount Hutt, Fox, Haast and Mount Cook). All had their charms, but I had a real soft spot for Blenheim.

When I first started doing medicals at Blenheim in 2002, I used the Marlborough Aero Club rooms at Omaka Airfield. But Stuart Tantrum offered me the use of a space in his new hangar and office complex, and in April I flew down to Omaka to catch up with Stu and check it out. I knew Stu from Foxton, where he had been based before he shifted south. He had always promised me he would set his new office up with an examination couch in anticipation of my arrival, and he was as good as his word. It was good while it lasted there, as his hangar was filled with beautifully restored First World War aircraft. Stu was a master craftsman.

When Stu succumbed to a long illness in 2011, I moved the NSRBFDS operation back into the Aero Club, this time using the old club rooms. Now this is one classy joint, with old native timber floors, a wall of piccies of aviation legend Charles Kingsford Smith from one of his visits in the 1930s, and a full 180-degree view of the airstrip, which meant I could keep an eye on who and what was flying. There are some really unique aircraft flying at Omaka. I remember once working away on my notes as some pilot was pulling up his trousers when I heard the 'chug chug chug' of an unfamiliar aircraft engine. I looked up and my jaw dropped as a Focke-Wulf FW 190 — a German fighter from the Second World War, tellingly nicknamed the Butcher Bird — taxied on past. Now that's something you don't see every day! Then there's Bill Reid's Avro Anson, a British twin-engined bomber also from the Second World War. I once managed to scrounge a few minutes flying as pilot in command of this thing; it chugged along at 90 knots over the coast of Marlborough, and it brought home to me what cannon fodder these light bombers had been, flying at 5000 feet over well-defended German positions.

In other words, for your aviation freak, Omaka is paradise, even without the Omaka Aviation Heritage Centre and its awesome displays, including Manfred von Richthofen's (otherwise known as the 'Red Baron') collection, which is owned by Sir Peter Jackson.

The other reason Omaka is extra special to me is because I have managed to rekindle old relationships with former Marlborough

Boys' College kids who, like me, somehow evaded the criminal justice system and went on to become fellow aviators — good bastards, such as Rex Newman and Ray Patchett. And with the NSRBFDS pretty much guaranteed to bring me into close contact with like-minded individuals, I have since developed many other great buddies down that way, too, including Willie Sage, Craig Anderson, Pete Anderson, Chris Brown, Geoff Van Asch, Graham and Jane Orphan, the Nimmos and Frank Prouting, to mention but a few. With these people I share the same love of the mountains and flying.

Motueka is another special place for me. I started doing aviation medicals there early on in 2001 at the Motueka Aerospace Research Centre. Motueka is beautiful, with its own micro-climate. It remains clear and dry while the rest of New Zealand suffers under a strong, southwesterly flow. But what really makes Motueka special to me are its people; great people like Giles and Katrina Witney and Jeremy Anderson of Nelson Aviation College, Andy Gillatt, Sid Deaker, Jim McGuire, Stu Bean and more. Penny Mackay, a previous owner of Nelson Aviation College, has been really good to Marc and me over the years, not only as a sounding board on aviation matters, but also as a bit of a mentor who has helped me deal with some of the slightly stranger bastards I have been involved with.

In the early days of doing medicals at Motueka, I also used to pop in to see Captain Bob Guard, who ran Air Nelson at the time. Now he's a man who could tell a tale or two! His great-grandfather was John Guard, who single-handedly confronted Te Rauparaha and his men for nicking his sheep — now that takes balls of steel! Bob himself had enormous aviation experience and was the co-pilot on the SAFE Air Armstrong Whitworth AW.660 Argosy that was involved in the famous Kaikoura UFO sighting in 1978. Bob always looks at the red strips on the top surface of my aircraft's wings and narrows his eyes at me.

Another bloke I keep going back to see is my old buddy and lawyer, Nick Davidson, whose world view seems to have been constructed from the pages of the satirical magazine *Punch*. I just love arguing politics and big-picture stuff over a coffee with Nick. No subject is too big or too sacred to escape his dry wit.

Special places, special people. It's what the NSRBFDS is all about.

Once, when I had finished doing medicals at Motueka, I popped in on Colin and Tina Nimmo at their place way up the Clarence River. The Nimmos' Muzzle Station is vast — over 100,000 acres — and because it is sandwiched between the parallel Inland and Seaward Kaikoura ranges, it is one of the hardest properties in New Zealand to reach. They run sheep, cattle and bees, and getting to and from and around the station involves lots of aircraft, both fixed-wing and helicopters.

On this occasion, I had done Colin's medical and I couldn't help noticing a huge set of deer antlers outside the door of their house, which was the original homestead of what was once Bluff Station.

'Shit, they're huge!' I exclaimed, fondling the velvet. A set of antlers like this are every hunter's dream trophy.

Colin dug his hands in his pockets and rounded his shoulders, striking the regulation pose for the delivery of a long and suspect yarn.

'Yeah, that thing was up that way, up a gully near the southern boundary . . .' he said. 'I stalked it here . . . blah blah . . . and there . . . blah blah . . .'

I was in the palm of his hand. Even allowing for the essential bit of fluffing up, this was plainly one of the epics of New Zealand deerstalking.

'. . . and then, at about 900 metres, it had to slow down to get through this narrow gap between two rocks and . . .'

Suddenly, Tina burst out of the door of the house.

'Bullshit, Colin,' she snapped. 'The bloody thing was in the orchard eating my apples, and I said, "Colin, if you don't go down there and shoot that thing, I'm leaving you." So he went down there and shot it from about 25 yards. So there!'

Once Marc and I had set up the infrastructure for the NSRBFDS on the West Coast, at Omarama and Aoraki/Mount Cook, we decided that was it. But as word spread about our very user-friendly service, the pressure from pilots ramped up to set up shop even further south. That would mean crossing the Alps a couple more times per trip and it's rare to get a long spell of perfect weather in that environment. It would also mean a lot more time and energy. I resisted, for a while.

But eventually, Toby Wallis and Morgie Saxton twisted my arm. Toby is a son of the legendary Sir 'Hurricane Tim' Wallis, who pioneered not only helicopter deer shooting and live recovery, but also the deer-farming industry and — for a hobby — the Warbirds movement, dedicated to the preservation and restoration of vintage warplanes. Toby was running Alpine Helicopters, the company that Tim set up. I already knew Morgie well, and after a few months of being badgered by this pair to nick through the Haast Pass every month and do a few medicals in Wanaka, I finally thought, what the heck. I duly established the Wanaka Aerospace Research Centre in the old Alpine Helicopters hangar, which was great for hangaring the aircraft overnight. As an added bonus it was also stuffed full of deer-hunting memorabilia and it helped, too, that my old buddies Uncle Keith and Aunt Jean lived close by, so Marc and I could generally stay with them.

I decided, then, that you may as well be hung for mutton as for lamb. One of the old-time pilots even further down the line at Te Anau rang me up to say there was a stack of pilots down there who wanted their medicals done. I've had a soft spot for Te Anau ever since my GP training days, of course, so I didn't have too much trouble saying yes.

Marc and I flew over and landed at the old Waiau airstrip to find a dozen pilots all standing around a barbecue ready for their medicals to be done. They were a good bunch, and all in that 'shark in the park' mood. I was in my element.

I'd emerge from doing a medical and someone would thrust a

plate of crayfish tails and sausages at me. I'd hold up my hands. 'Better not. Gotta wash my hands first. Doug's got gonorrhoea.'

'I knew it! So have half his sheep!' someone would yell.

'Lucky bastard,' someone else would say. 'At least it means he's getting some.'

Once I'd done the work, we would load the gear in the aircraft along with a heap of crayfish tails, some malt vinegar as dressing, a full coffee flask and head back home. We'd get back to Palmy so stuffed with crayfish that we could hardly get out of the plane.

The other beauty of flying in to Te Anau regularly is that it always soothes the lingering pangs of regret I've had ever since I turned down the chance to live and work there permanently.

I quickly came to appreciate that it's quite a dangerous place to fly in the winter. The Te Anau basin has a tendency to collect low cloud and fog, and I'm sure it's killed its share of pilots over the years. There has been more than one occasion where I have set off from Palmy in a beautiful, clear predawn with the weather map showing a huge anticyclone draped over the South Island.

One time I travelled the full distance and had four hours' flying on autopilot at 10,000 feet, until the very last phase of the flight, where I crossed the Routeburn Track and the Hollyford Valley. I was feeling pretty relaxed by this point, after watching a beautiful sunrise and spending a lot of time glassing the mountaintops for chamois and deer. But then, 45 nautical miles north of Te Anau, when I passed over the last range of mountains that form the northern rim of the Te Anau basin . . .

'Shit! SHIT!'

The whole basin was filled with a thick layer of low-lying stratus cloud with the tops at about 3000 feet. The cloud base might have been hugging the ground in a soupy fog or holding 500 feet above it — there was no way of knowing. Typically, I would descend and skim over the cloud top, keeping my fingers crossed that Waiau would be clear. If I fly over the Waiau airstrip and Te Anau township without seeing any suspicion of a hole in the cloud, I've often been obliged to carry on south to where there's often a hole up around Lake Manapouri or at the head of the Iris Burn River.

If I spotted a hole, I'd breathe a sigh of relief and work my way down beneath the cloud base about 600 feet above the lake. Then I'd slow the aircraft down into what is called poor weather configuration, setting 10 degrees of flap and the engine power to 20 inches/2400 RPM so I would have more time to make decisions. The dangerous bit is the approach to the airstrip through patches of fog that are hugging the ground. It can suddenly close in on you from behind so you're trapped.

In a helicopter, you can just pop down into a small clearing in the bush, but fixed-wing aircraft need lots of room to land. Most of the time, before the Waiau airstrip was closed in 2009, I got in under these conditions, and landed with my heart still thumping. Other times, it just didn't seem right, so I would pull out and either spend an hour tiki-touring around the Fiordland National Park waiting for the cloud to lift, or fly the short distance to land at Mossburn, where I could wait for things to clear, or just refuel and bugger off if it didn't.

A mate of mine, Bob Cleland, has occasionally made his place at Mossburn available to me to use for medicals, and that has worked out OK, as it's not too long a journey for everyone to drive up from Te Anau. But whatever . . . I must have made the right decisions so far, because I am still alive to tell the tale.

After the Waiau airstrip closed, I was forced to move operations to the very flash new Te Anau Airport Manapouri. It's a great airport and the take-off roll, heading to the west and looking out over Lake Manapouri to the mountains, has to be one of the most beautiful in the world. But when I can, I prefer to use either the Upukerora Aerospace Research Institute or the Milford Sound Aerospace Research Unit.

=

I established the Upukerora Aerospace Research Institute at Sid 'Noddy' Deaker's place just north of Te Anau. It was Noddy's brother, Dick, who invited me in the first place. Dick has been a licensed pilot for more than 50 years, which is all the more remarkable given that most of his flying has been done in the helicopter deer-recovery business. You'll sometimes hear people say that there are old helicopter pilots and bold helicopter pilots, but no old, bold helicopter pilots. Dick is perhaps unique, because he's carried the colossal gonads that chopper boys have as a breed into advanced age. For much of that time, Noddy has been Dick's shooter, and he is renowned for having shot over 100,000 deer.

The Deakers' hangar, where I have my clinic, oozes history. It used to be the maintenance facility for a number of small aviation outfits that carried out various activities around Fiordland National Park. One of the walls is covered with old photos that have backed me up every time someone has accused me of being a blouse for refusing to fly to Big Bay (also known as Awarua

Bay). Big Bay is a scoop out of the rugged West Coast located about 30 nautical miles north of Milford Sound. It's surrounded by lofty, bush-clad peaks and, being so remote and inaccessible, it's a paradise for hunting, shooting, fishing types, many of whom prefer to fly in rather than trudge in on foot or risk that exposed bit of coastline to go in by sea. There are no real technical aviation challenges involved in getting there: the only problem is that the landing strip is the beach. Call me fussy, but I've never liked the thought of exposing the fuselage of my little plane to the corrosive effects of salt water, and besides, it's a bit of a skill knowing how to taxi an aircraft up into the sand dunes without getting stuck. And there is an entire wall of photos at Upukerora that attest to the fact that if you fuck up a beach landing, you'll more than likely hit soft sand and tip over, whereupon the tide will come in and deliver the *coup de grâce*.

But I have no such reservations about flying in to Milford Sound. Even though it's one of New Zealand's most visited tourist attractions, Milford Sound still retains a raw, untouched beauty. It doesn't matter if you fly in via any of the many mountain passes or by sea, the sight of its steep mountains rearing straight out of the mirror-calm sound is mind-blowing. The more I fly in to this place, the more I get off on it. The Milford Sound Aerospace Research Unit is located in Jeff Shanks' hangar and it's an amazing place to stay overnight. Marc and I used to wander out and look at the blaze of the Milky Way and the hard glitter of the stars, and we'd have no doubt that our lucky ones were somewhere up there amongst them.

CHAPTER 10

MATURING AS AN ORGANISATION

As I approached the strip at Haast one beautiful morning, I noted a couple of horses strolling around. I did a low pass or two to encourage them to move on, and when the coast was clear, I lined up and put ZK-Really-Jolly-Good down. As I taxied over to my usual parking spot, I saw that the Wallis family's Cessna 180 was parked on the airstrip, too. That meant Toby had flown Sir Tim — who was no longer medically fit to fly, after one air crash too many — over to see Dave Saxton for a cuppa. I was on more than nodding terms with Sir Tim. I'd quite often see him in the Wanaka hangar and would have a chat with this gentlemanly legend of New Zealand aviation.

The clatter of a Hughes 500D announced the arrival of Morgie to pick me up from the airstrip. After setting my gear up in the Haast Aerospace Research Centre, I did five or six aviation medical examinations as per usual. When I finished, I looked in to the house to see if the Saxtons and Wallises were about for a chat. They seemed to have buggered off somewhere, so I chucked my stuff into one of Dave's jeeps and drove back to the strip.

It turned out that's where everyone was. They were all assembled around the jeep Sir Tim was sitting in and having a big old bullshit session. I pulled up next to ZK-Really-Jolly-Good to drop my gear off and immediately spotted a big dent in the lower left cowl of the nose of the aircraft.

'What the fuck caused that?' I cursed loudly.

The meeting around Sir Tim's vehicle dissolved and reconvened around ZK-Really-Jolly-Good, where much scratching of heads ensued. A bit of snorting and stamping from the far end of the airstrip gave the game away.

'That bloody nag of Debbie's!' said Dave.

A quick glance at the dent confirmed it was a good fit for the hind hoof of a mongrel brumby hell-bent on vengeance.

'Mustn't have liked being shooed off the runway,' I muttered.

'You prize prick!' shouted Dave at the horse. 'I'll get you for this!'

Five hundred metres downrange, the horse tossed its mane and whinnied. It sounded suspiciously like it was laughing at us.

Conversation then turned to whether it was safe to fly the aircraft home for repairs. The accumulated hours and combined knowledge of the group of five pilots present was immense, and debate raged for the better part of 10 minutes. Then Morgan suggested we ask what Sir Tim thought. Everyone nodded and without further ado, Toby fetched the jeep in which Sir Tim was sitting 50 metres away and drove right up close to the front of my plane.

Sir Tim studied the damage out of the window as everyone held their breath. It was like all of those times I'd spent on ward rounds with a cluster of junior doctors awaiting the pronouncement of an esteemed consultant.

After a minute or so, Sir Tim simply said: 'It's safe.' Everyone looked at one another, shrugged their shoulders and nodded. The matter was settled and everyone walked away from my dented aircraft. That's the kind of esteem in which Sir Tim Wallis is held.

They're good bastards in the Deep South. Good bastards, but occasionally dangerous bastards, too — a danger to themselves and to others. A couple of stories will serve to illustrate the point.

Once upon a time, there was a high-country farmer who owned a pastoral lease over a certain block high in the Southern Alps. Besides his sheep, there were a fair number of deer running around on the land. As leaseholder, our man — let's call him Bill, to protect the innocent — assumed he owned the deer, too, and got to say who turned up with a rifle to have a crack at them.

Anyone who tried potting a deer on someone's farm without their permission was a poacher.

Until the mid-1960s, Bill's world view went largely unchallenged. But not even high-country farmers can stop progress, and the arrival of the helicopter changed everything. Along with the proliferation of choppers, there arose a new, free-spirited breed of bloke with big balls and a corresponding lack of regard for life and limb. It occurred to these men that all those nice fat deer bouncing around in the hills represented a vast, untapped resource just waiting to be harvested by anyone with a rifle and balls big enough to do it. After all, the New Zealand government owned the land, dinnit, and therefore the deer were public property.

You can sort of see where this was going. The first commercial helicopter flight for the purpose of shooting deer happened in 1964, and after that, it was all on. When the price of venison went through the roof in the early 1970s, choppers began buzzing around the tops like Jackson Bay sandflies around a nudist on a muggy day. Thousands of deer were shot off high-country pastureland, while outraged cockies like Bill watched helplessly through binos and, every so often, telescopic sights. Eventually the air force had to be called in to try to cool down what became known as the 'helicopter wars'.

It all simmered down eventually, with live deer recovery and deer farming taking the place of wild harvest, but the bad blood that accumulated during that period lingered on — as I was to find out.

Nearly three decades on from when it all took place, Bill — no doubt older, wiser, sadder — invited me to drop in on him for breakfast en route from Haast to the Queenstown Lakes District. I accepted with pleasure: he'd lived in a fabulous part of the country for decades and was bound to have some good stories to tell.

The night before, I finished all my medicals and joined Dave and Debbie Saxton, who were putting me up, for a bite of dinner. I was sitting there, beer in hand, as Debbie loaded up my plate with meat and veges.

'Whatcha got planned for tomorrow, Doc?' asked Dave, as he reached for his own beer.

'I've got a breakfast date over the way,' I replied.

'Oh, yeah. Who?'

A slight, premonitory chill ran down my spine. I knew enough about the history in these parts to know what farmers like Bill thought of chopper pilots like Dave, even if I had always scrupulously refrained from taking sides in the old argument.

'Oh, some bloke. Can't really remember his name,' I fudged desperately.

'Come on. You're having breakfast with the bastard. You must remember his name,' Dave said sceptically.

'Oh, it's . . . Bill,' I said, and mumbled the surname, not meeting Dave's eye. The temperature dropped abruptly. I glanced up at Dave and saw that his face had turned red and his eyes had gone all squinty and evil-like. He was gripping the table with white knuckles.

'That fucken bastard!' he roared, and started to get to his feet, still holding the heavy table so that it tilted and everything began to slide off. 'You're visiting that prick?'

'Cut it out, Dave!' Debbie yelled, trying to trim the table by leaning her full weight on the high side.

'Don't tell me who to be friends with, Dave,' I said. 'Or I'm outta here.'

Debbie gave him a good dressing-down which included a lot of yelling and wild gyrations of the upper limbs. Dave still wasn't happy, though, and filled me in good and proper on the history and exactly why he thought Bill was a prize prick. Once it was off his chest, he went back to his usual colour and we resumed laughing and telling each other fluffed-up stories.

The next day I was up well before daybreak and, after a cuppa, I got ZK-Really-Jolly-Good preflighted and ready to go. While I waited for daylight I gazed at the huge, bright, full moon that hangs over Haast and marvelled at how it looked as though you could almost touch it. When the first rays of sunlight arrived, I got myself airborne and headed for my breakfast date.

It was a beautiful, clear, frosty morning so it didn't take long to skip through the mountains and find Bill's farm airstrip. I knew he was a bit deaf so I did a low pass over his farmhouse before landing to let him know I was there. By the time I was on the ground and killing the motor, he had turned up in a beat-up old jeep. He was immaculately dressed, his white hair neatly combed, and he greeted me with a firm handshake and plenty of old-school charm. We drove the couple of kilometres to his lovely little country cottage where I was introduced to his friendly, smiling wife. Both of them were very hospitable and I was soon sipping coffee next to their pussycat curled up by their open fire with the smell of bacon and eggs cooking on the old stove wafting through the room.

Bill and I were duly summoned to take our places at the

beautifully laid table and as we sat down, he politely asked where I had stayed the night before.

Oh, shit. I had that chill again.

'Oh, just with a mate,' I said casually.

'Oh, yes,' he persisted. 'Do you mind me asking who?'

'Oh, you know. A mate. A good bastard. A really good bastard, old Sax . . .' I coughed as I said the name, in the hope that he wouldn't hear it.

'Saxton,' Bill said the name flatly. 'Saxton? You stayed with DAVE SAXTON?'

He went from debonair country gent to roaring maniac in the space of a heartbeat, his face twisted with demonic fury, his eyes protruding and veins throbbing visibly in his temples. He lifted his side of the table and fine china and silver cutlery crashed to the floor.

'Bill!' his wife shrieked. 'For God's sake, cut it out!'

I swear he would have gone for me had his wife not grabbed the back of his collar and pulled on it so hard his jugular veins poked out. His face went from scarlet to a funny shade of blue, but his arms were still stretched out towards me, his fingers twitching in the direction of my throat. There was a bang as their cat hit the cat flap at 100 knots.

His wife dragged old Bill by the collar to a distant room in the house and for 10 minutes they screamed at each other with no regard at all for my tender, innocent ears. I took the opportunity to grab some toast from the kitchen bench and scraped a bit of scrambled egg off the floor. All the excitement was making me hungry.

I was about to hightail it the same way as the cat had, but they both suddenly reappeared. There was an uneasy pause while Bill's missus looked at him expectantly.

'I think we'd best change the subject,' Bill gritted.

Good bloody idea, I thought, but didn't dare say so.

Bill's missus then asked me to sit down by the fire again, which I did rather nervously, and they quickly cleaned the place up. Once order was restored, we moved on and got talking on a variety of topics, such as the state of high-country farming and flying in the Alps. It all turned out really good and the food was none the worse for having spent a bit of time on the kitchen floor. When I left, they waved goodbye as though nothing had happened. I took off scratching my head as to how such really good people on both sides could make such dicks of themselves about stuff that happened 20 years ago.

'A bit of Zen Buddhism wouldn't go astray down here,' I mumbled to myself as I levelled ZK-Really-Jolly-Good off at a cruise 24/24 power setting, at which she performs her best.

—

On another occasion, when I was driving due to poor weather and after I had overnighted at Hoki, I had the bright idea of dropping in on Pete 'the Bushman' Salter at Pukekura, just down the road. I knew four o'clock in the morning was a bit early in most people's books, so there would be risks.

The first was getting down to Pete and Justine's house along an overgrown pathway in the pitch-black of a moonless, West Coast night. Unfortunately, my torch was busted so I lit a match every five metres to keep me on track. It took a good 15 minutes and a full box of matches to make it down the path.

The second risk was getting past their trusty guard dog. That was easy, because I've found over the years that 99 per cent of guard dogs are partial to half a roll of salami. Pete and Justine's dog was not one of the one per cent. With that mission accomplished and happy sounds of munching coming from behind me, I strode up to the back door, banged on it good and loud, went in and flicked on the light.

There were a few thumps and grunts from upstairs, and then the wholly unanticipated risk three appeared, in the form of a largely naked Pete emerging from the darkened stairwell brandishing a monstrous knife.

'Who the fuck's that?' he rasped.

'Pete!' I squeaked. 'It's me! Hey, it's me! You know, Dave — your good mate Dave. Remember me? Dave? Dave the Pacifist . . .'

To my great relief, after rubbing his eyes a bit, he recognised me and put the rather sharp pointy thing down. I was lucky Pete had the sense to ask questions first! As my heart rate returned to normal, I wished I'd had a camera to capture an image of this extra-hairy, Neanderthal-looking bushman, almost as nude as the day he was born. He was lucky I wasn't a sheila: I might have been turned on!

After we had been yarning for a few minutes, risk number four became apparent. Justine had been cowering under the covers the whole time, fearing the worst, and when she eventually realised I wasn't some raping, burgling home invader, her thoughts turned to vengeance. The bollocking only lasted a minute or so and before long the coffee was on and we were having a laugh about it all.

All was forgiven — of me at least. I'm not sure how the dog got on when Pete took up the matter of how easily he could be bribed to keep quiet with just half a roll of salami.

I had pretty much always resisted the idea of taking in a partner at the Bulls Medical Centre. By the middle of 2002, though, it was pretty obvious that there was only so much Dr Dave to go around. I was still working four days a week at the medical centre and building up the Bulls Flying Doctor Service, at the same time as trying to operate it as well.

One day, Sandi and I were at The Portage in the Marlborough Sounds where I was attending a medical conference. We were having a walk, and discussing how there just weren't enough hours in the day for me to get everything done. Sandi suggested I consider sharing the medical centre and I was just in the process of agreeing with her when who should materialise before me but Dr Ken Young and his wife Lesley. Dr Ken and I got talking. He was running the medical centre up the road in Taihape and was every bit as burnt out as me. He and Lesley had just been talking about maybe moving to a larger centre, which would be good for their young children, and would also give Dr Ken the chance to fulfil a wish to go back to school and study sports medicine.

It was as though I had conjured my fairy godmother (although in my imagination, my fairy godmother features less facial hair and doesn't have a Glaswegian accent). Either way, it felt like synchronicity. Between the four of us, we decided that the

MATURING AS AN ORGANISATION

Youngs would be mad if they didn't shift to Palmy, where Ken could study sports medicine at Massey, and their kids could go to a bigger and better school. Ken could help me out by filling in as a locum, with a view to coming aboard in a more meaningful way down the track.

So that's exactly what happened. One year later, in mid-2003, once I'd had the chance to confirm my initial impressions that Ken was in the same hard-working, good-looking mould as myself, Ken formally bought into the practice. It was a major development because he had the kind of fancy, fresh ideas about computers and developing new systems that every practice needs. His enthusiasm was like a breath of fresh air for me and just about every idea he came up with — with the notable exception that we should move some of my model aircraft — was easy to say yes to. The practice went ahead in leaps and bounds, and this allowed me more time and space to devote to the NSRBFDS.

By this point, I owned Bulls Medical Centre outright and it had been easiest for NSRBFDS to be based there. All of the administration gear and pilot notes were kept either in a back room called 'The Lab' or up at the Skunk Works at RNZAF Base Ohakea.

I was spending long hours at the medical centre doing regular daily clinics as well as frequent weekends and nights on call, which meant sleeping on the premises. 'The Lab' came in handy for this, too. Karen Greer, our extraordinarily wonderful manager, handled the NSRBFDS administration work and this became an increasingly significant demand on her time.

The combination of having the two companies under one roof at Bulls, and having the hangar facilities next door to the well-appointed military base down the road had been perfect. But in fairness to Ken, I really had to create some separation between the medical centre and the NSRBFDS.

The time felt ripe anyway. In the wake of the terrorist attacks on 11 September 2001, things had begun to change at Ohakea. The attitude towards the civilian community shifted in light of the perceived need for increased security. Ex-staff and locals who'd long been associated with the base and could use the pool and other facilities, now came to be seen as 'security risks' and were prohibited from entering the base. It was a real shame; in no time the tight bond between the community and the base, which had been built over many, many years, broke down. If they'd stopped to think about it, they would have realised that all that goodwill out there in the local community was a much more effective guarantor of the base's security than all of the over-zealous security guards they could have hired. It's only in recent years that they seem to have started to try to repair the damage.

I began to feel unwelcome myself, and when I drove around, I noticed big white security vehicles with red lights on top followed me. Marc and I occasionally had a bit of a giggle leading them on a wild goose chase around the base and then hiding in someone's garage to watch them whizz by us all in a lather. But as the numbers of pilots coming to me for their medicals increased, so did the need to provide convenient aerial access for them. With things at Ohakea going the way they were, it was pretty obvious that a new home was needed for the NSRBFDS.

Moving was going to cost a lot of time and money, so we needed to make sure we got it right. Marc was vitally involved in the decision-making, because by now, not only was he helping with the NSRBFDS, but he was also close to realising his ambition of getting his commercial helicopter pilot licence and setting up his own business flying choppers.

Talking it over, we decided that what was needed was a purpose-built aviation medical centre with hangarage for ZK-Really-Jolly-Good and room to park a chopper, too. The first challenge was to sort out the best airport; it needed to be well-lit and offer 24-hour IFR flying. This ruled out Feilding and Pine Park. Whanganui was a possibility, but all things considered, it was obvious we'd be mad if we didn't try for Palmy. It answered all of our requirements and, as it turned out, airport manager Gary Goodman and his mates were so friendly and helpful that our choice ended up being a very happy one. We were allocated an awesome spot right next to the control tower, security and fuel facilities, for which we were eternally grateful. The site was also close to Massey's School of Aviation, which was established in the late 1980s and was now moving ahead. The proximity offered us the opportunity to develop a relationship with a stimulating and motivated university aviation department. I grabbed it with both hands.

With the location sorted, now all we needed was the dosh. We set up cookie stalls around the Manawatu to raise money for our new venture, but when sales proved poor, we had to do a grovelly for a loan to our good mates Lynley Rogers and Martin Stokes in the Medical Assurance Society. They were obliging as ever, so a few signatures later it was all systems go for the Palmy headquarters of the NSRBFDS.

The builder in our family, cuzzy-bro Richard, set to work designing and building the new facility, but we needed somewhere to store our shit in the meantime. Help came locally and we were very grateful to local chopper pilot Rick Lucas for lending us one of his empty hangars, and to Bill Olsen at Fieldair, who made some of his office space available to us for pilot medical examinations.

After notifying the RNZAF we were moving out of Ohakea — they could hardly conceal their relief and joy — we moved out of Skunk Works and not without regret. It was the end of an era, although I gather the legend lives on: the hangar is still known amongst airmen who weren't born when I first set up there as 'Dr Dave's'. I relocated the administrative side of the NSRBFDS to the little office I have at home, and I deposited all the pilot notes and records in a shed out the back where we also keep the lawnmower and sacks of onions and spuds. You can imagine how impressed the CAA medical team were by this arrangement when they came to do my first audit!

Moving was a real mission, but it was also exciting. It was a quantum leap forward in how the NSRBFDS would work and the potential development of the business was enormous. But more importantly, it also offered the prospect of deepening my relationship with Marc.

At this time Marc was intensively working to get his chopper licence. Under the tuition of Mike Bryant at Flight Training Manawatu, Marc soloed in a fixed-wing late in 2003 (when he was 16) and got his PPL a year later. He completed his chopper licence soon afterwards and did his full IFR rating and fixed-wing CPL in quick succession. The only hiccup in his march through the successive stages of advanced aviation competency came when he got the flu and developed an acute viral infection of the heart. Luckily, between Dr Ken at Bulls Medical Centre and Dr Malcolm Abernethy — Camellia's old bedmate — he was fixed up with no lasting damage. At the point where the Palmerston North Aerospace Research Centre (as we christened it) was nearing completion at the end of its six-month construction period, we were leasing a Robinson R22 so that he could build up his hours.

To pick up the NSRBFDS admin work that Marc had been doing (Karen had left when Dr Ken came on board), we hired Jean Adams, known as Flying Jeanie, to help. Flying Jeanie was an ex-prison guard, and proved to be very efficient as an administrator. She got on well with the pilots and commanded a lot of respect from them, because she sure as hell didn't take any shit.

=

On 20 December 2005, a big crowd — including Dave Saxton, Harvey Hutton and Dick Deaker from the Deep South and, of course, Granny Olive, who was never one to miss a party — gathered for the formal opening of the Palmerston North Aerospace Research Centre by John Jones, the director of the Civil Aviation Safety Authority. Right from the laying of the first foundation stone I was determined this facility would have a spiritual dimension to it. I figured a combination of Maori and run-of-the-mill honky Christian religious stuff that I favour would do the trick. The front of the hangar proudly displays a maihi, which was carved for us specially out of totara that came from the Rangitikei River near Bulls. On either side of the maihi is a kowhaiwhai pattern representing kawakawa leaves, which are revered by Maori for their healing qualities. When the building was completed, I had a Rangitane minister bless it, and at the opening ceremony, I had both a Maori elder and a minister of the church pronounce their blessings on it. And then, with the formalities over, we were open for business!

The first customers turned up for their medicals the very next day, and we didn't look back. Our location made it easy for pilots to get to us, whether travelling by road or air. And with time, the facilities have had various additions, such as a purpose-built communications room fully loaded with computers and the best satellite, VHF and UHG-HF equipment around. So whizz-bang is our set-up that we've put it at the disposal of the police as a back-up base for local search and rescue operations.

Looking back now, I see that those were golden years. Marc and I were both flat out with our own jobs — Marc working towards his dream of establishing his own helicopter operation, and me working three days a week in the Bulls Medical Centre — and we also had the monster that was our shared project, the NSRBFDS.

With any job, even a dream one like the NSRBFDS, routines form. This means the random events, where we end up doing strange things in strange places, become the highlights of trips and form memories that are never to be forgotten.

I reckon the dodgiest place I ever did a pilot medical was in a chicken coop up near the Rakaia River. It really was one to remember: I had this bloke laid out on a bench amongst the nest boxes while I did an echocardiogram (ECG), as a few dozen chooks clucked and flapped and eyed the machine's little screen curiously. Every now and then I had to brush one of the cloud of feathers flying around the place off the equipment. Despite chook poo on his clothes, the client was grateful because I'd managed to squeeze his urgent medical into my already frantic schedule.

Then, of course, there was that *other* time when I was at Pete the Bushman's place at Pukekura to do a medical for my old mate John Kerr, who happened to be driving through at the same time. A suitable facility was hard to find: John's a big bugger and being very conscious of health and safety, I was worried the tables in the local café might not be up to the job. I eventually settled on the bar in Pete and Justine's establishment. John wasn't so keen, but I managed to convince him to stop moaning and lie down.

'There's no one around,' I told him. 'It'll only take a jiff.'

Grumbling, John eventually consented to take off his shirt and recline on the bar. I wired him up with the ECG leads, with the assistance of gorgeous Nurse Pete Salter. We tried not to giggle at the sight of him, lying semi-naked on the bar, festooned with wires and his moderately big potbelly rising and falling in time with his heavy, anxious breathing. Everything was trucking along fine when, out of the blue, we heard the hiss of air brakes outside.

'Well, I'll be damned,' I said.

'Fucken hurry up!' yelled John, but it was too late. The room was already filling up with German tourists exclaiming loudly in German.

'Blitzer und Donner!'

'Mein Gott!'

'Was ist das, Herr Doktor?'

The more inquisitive and medically aware formed a tightly packed group around John on the bar, and I began to get the uneasy feeling that John might be about to become a social media star in Germany. John tried to get up but as he was all wired up, I had to yell at him to keep still so I could finish the ECG recording.

'Ja, is best to keep schtill,' a tourist opined, and others nodded sagely. Pete and Justine were pissing themselves with laughter. John darted me a murderous look, but stayed still long enough to finish the ECG. When at last I allowed him to get up, he swore that this would be the first and last time he was medically examined on a bar. Auf wiedersehen, John boy!

Life, in short, was seldom dull. And best of all, Marc was usually along for the ride when I had these adventures, and we laughed and laughed. Even when he wasn't, he was the ideal audience on which to practise my slightly embellished versions of these stories. Life was good.

… CHAPTER 11 …

A FEW WEST COAST TALES

The Gang of Three were all quietly buzzing. It was April. There was a fine dusting of snow on the tops of the Alps, but the weather forecast was excellent and the new day was colouring in the sky with a big blue crayon.

We were heading for the Maori Lakes, which are a bunch of large alpine tarns high on the easternmost spur of the Olivine Range. My favourite of these is Lake Leeb, which is the highest of them all. This area is one of the most beautiful alpine places to explore from the air, with its wide open tops and perfect views of the surrounding mountains, the water of the lakes shading from emerald to tawny brown and the surrounding landscape pleasantly pleated and covered with lush, green bush. It's a deerstalker's paradise, with lots of deer and long ridges of open bush making for easy walking.

Morgan Saxton arrived in his chopper.

'Just another shitty day,' he observed, as he began loading our gear. This would take a while, because as everyone in these parts knew by now, the Baldwins didn't travel light. We liked our home comforts, we did, and you try separating Granny Olive from her beloved camp oven.

Once we were all loaded up, Morgie's machine heaved into the air and rose towards the mountains. I caught Marc's eye and he gave me an excited thumbs up. This was going to be fucking great.

Over the next few days, Marc and I hunted around the lakes. After a while, we began focusing our attention on a large open, grassy flat around a pair of small tarns, as there seemed to be a very big stag living in the area. It was making a shit-load of noise. Several times we got quite close to it, but just as we thought we were going to get a crack at it, it would suddenly go all quiet on us. The flats in question were a good couple of hours from base camp, so Marc and I decided if we were going to be serious about nailing this particular animal, we'd best fly-camp in the area so that we'd be there with time on our hands in the evening and at first light.

We loaded up our packs with overnight gear and said our farewells to Granny Olive. Far from being fazed, she loved the idea of spending the night alone in this place with two bottles of bubbly and her old conquest, Tititea/Mount Aspiring, looming to the south, a reminder of her youth and vigour. We set off down the ridge. Twenty minutes of solid walking later, we could still hear her yodelling away behind us, and I could picture her standing pirouetting in the tussock, like some antipodean version of Julie Andrews in *The Sound of Music*.

Just before we reached the bushline, there was the sudden whining roar of a turbine engine and a Hughes 300 rose over the ridge and set down. The door opened and there was Dave Sax holding out a roast chook. We were rapt with the chook, but Dave also saved us a couple of hours of walking with heavy packs. He dropped us at the flat where we were heading and that meant more hunting time for the boys!

As soon as the chopper had gone, we quickly set up camp and took advantage of the extra hour's daylight we now had available to us by heading off for an evening shoot. We walked up to the head of one of the small lakes, working our way through the open bush that surrounded a small creek that fed into the lake. We were traipsing along quietly when the alpine silence was broken by a loud, reverberating roar.

We both jumped in fright. Not only was it close, but the stag sounded really mean! In fact, it sounded decidedly pissed off. We could hear our own hearts thumping as we edged forward. We heard more roars and crashing about in the bush no more than 100 metres away. I looked at Marc and he looked back at me, grinning excitedly. His face was pale with fright, but it also had that 'Shit, this is awesome' look that I'm sure I was wearing, too.

Gradually we worked our way closer and closer until I reckoned we were about 30 metres from the stag, which was still thrashing about. The bush was just a little bit too thick for us to see him. I had the magazine in the rifle and the action half closed and ready, but there was no point in trying to get any closer. We'd just have to wait in the hope His Highness would pop out of the thicket and let us have a crack at him.

Minutes passed. There was crashing, banging and roaring in the bush ahead of us; it felt so close, like we could spit on the critter. But then there was an eerie silence that stretched into two or three minutes, then five. Still we waited, but there was simply nothing.

Marc and I looked at each other in disbelief and disappointment, but there was bugger all we could do about it. The stag had just disappeared into thin air — we didn't even hear him go! We sat down for a while to contemplate the situation and then, with no further sign of him, we got up and worked our way back to our fly-camp, grumbling and cursing all the way.

It was hard to stay mad when we got back to our fly-camp in the fading light of another crystal-clear mountain evening. We sat on tree stumps munching on our roast chook while looking out over the cool, grey expanse of the tussock flat, with the lake reflecting the last of the light. There was the prickle of settling dew and the inky blackness of the bush, and the first stars. We sucked away on them chicken bones and talked stratagems for getting that wretched stag in the morning. It was a moonless night, but the stars of the Milky Way shone flat and hard as diamonds. It was utterly still, apart from the odd squawk from the kea that lived in the area. Every now and then, we heard a husky roar from our mate on a distant ridge. These roars made us chuckle; we reckoned the bloody stag was laughing at us dumb-arse hunters who couldn't shoot jack shit.

Those couple of hours in that place — I don't know whether

I knew it at the time or whether I have imbued it with a special significance looking back, but I consider those to have been some of the happiest moments of my life. I had never felt closer to Marc or more at home in my own skin. I felt I was in the right place and in the best of all possible worlds. It's hard to know whether to remember that time with a sense of joy or loss. Some feelings are best simply felt, and not analysed or teased apart.

=

After another brew that night, we climbed into our sleeping bags. You're conscious of the chill and the dew over everything at first, but then your body heat warms up your bag and the pleasant ache of your tired leg muscles — and the sore ribs where you've been laughing too much — asserts itself and you drift off to sleep.

I think I dropped off imagining barrelling a monstrous stag in the very near future, but the next thing I remember was feeling with absolute certainty that I was falling into a big black hole and that I was going to die. It was horrible, and I've never experienced anything like it since. In the middle of it I was awoken by a tearing sound and a tremendous roar.

'Fuck!' I screamed. 'What was that?'

It was all but pitch-black, but when the tearing sound came again, I had a glimpse of the sky and made out the tent fly being torn off its guys and landing on top of Marc, who was struggling to get out of his sleeping bag.

'ROAR! ROAR!'

Trampling and stamping sounds boomed right next to my ear.

'Jesus!' yelled Marc.

'Yeah, Lord!' I yelled too. 'A little help here, too, please!'

By this time, I had fumbled my headlamp on. I grabbed my .270 and had chambered a round, still lying half in and half out of my sleeping bag. The stag was going mental, and to say I was feeling shit scared is an understatement. I aimed the rifle in the direction of the worst of the noise. The batteries in my headlamp were nearly flat so it cast only a feeble glow a couple of metres in front of me; with no focal point, I didn't have a hope in hell of getting a good sight of him.

The roaring seemed to have moved towards the clearing which was now moonlit. I wriggled out of my sleeping bag and crept along, parallel to the sound, in my undies and bare feet, but still pointing the rifle in the general direction of the noise in case the stag charged me. Marc was still tangled up in the tent fly and was making strange gargling noises as he tried to get free.

The tussock flat was beautifully clear in the starlight. I was hoping like hell that our mate would venture out of the cover of the bush and onto this flat so that I could get a shot at him. He didn't. At intervals he kept roaring in the impenetrable blackness under the trees, I swear no more than 20 metres from me. Then, after 10 minutes, everything went silent. It was a few minutes before he roared again, this time from quite a distance away.

'Fuck me,' I said to Marc, who had just got it together and joined me. 'The bastard dug us out of our camp.'

We looked at each other. He was in his undies, very white in the feeble beam of the headlamp, wide-eyed and shivering. I was in exactly the same state. I swung the beam back to our wrecked campsite.

'He did everything but shag us!' I said.

'We should be grateful for that, I suppose,' said Marc. 'We've still got our virginity.'

What do you do in a situation like that? Laugh? Cry? Recite poetry? Well, we laughed until we were fit to wet ourselves, and every time the stag roared in the distance, we laughed harder.

When we got back to base camp later that morning, Granny Olive listened intently to our tale, nodding seriously at our every word. After hearing us out in silence (which was unusual for her), she said: 'Well, I think that stag came up here last night, too.'

She leaned in towards us and lowered her voice to a spine-chilling whisper.

'When I went to the toilet in the dark last night,' she breathed, 'I was sure I was being followed. Thank goodness I had my knife on me.'

She paused for dramatic effect and fondled the hilt of her knife where it was tucked into her shorts.

'We need to be more careful, dear,' she hissed.

I looked at Marc. He looked back at me with wide, shiny eyes that laughed in the sunlight.

'Yup,' we said in unison, sharing a wink. 'Yes, Mum. We'll have to be very, very careful in future.'

Far from marauding stags, the Bulls Flying Doctor Service was taking off (to coin a phrase). I was acquiring more and more clients, and with the installation of a whizz-bang new database that would automatically generate lists of people who needed reminding that their medical was due and that they needed to make an appointment, my caseload was growing, too.

From time to time, the Flying Doctor became the Driving Doctor, usually because bad weather moved in down south when I had a full schedule of medicals to perform and to cancel would seriously inconvenience a whole lot of people. The terrestrial back-up involved the Interislander and my trusty Ford Ranger four-wheel drive complete with big tyres and spotlights.

I love driving nearly as much as I love flying, because it means I can stop off to visit old friends and check out interesting places that I'd previously spotted from the air and have a nosey around. Once I clocked an old campsite while flying through the Haast Pass; it was well off the road and it seemed likely that it was hardly ever visited. A month later, Marc and I were driving through Haast Pass and we allowed time to walk into this historic site. It turned out to be old accommodation for pioneers and their horses passing through what remains to this day a very rough piece of real estate. It was an authentic glimpse into the hard lives of the old-timers. After spending a couple of hours poking around, we took a few bits and pieces back to Palmy for our Aviation Medical Centre, including an old bullet-holed chimney.

Some of the stories we acquired while driving were just as fun to tell during long winter evenings as the tales we accumulated while flying. Once, when we were on our way up to the Mackenzie Basin to do a load of medicals up there, we stopped for a piss off the Rakaia Bridge. Marc was dreamily bleeding the lizard when there was a shout from below. He looked down to see a very grumpy looking kayaker waving his fist back up at him!

A FEW WEST COAST TALES

Now and again, and usually through stress of weather or because everyone has been too busy making the most of a fine spell at some remote location, it's been more convenient for the mountain to come to Muhammad, and I have arranged to meet groups of pilots at some random airstrip that I don't normally visit. Variety is the spice of life, as they say, and I've never minded.

One time we got to Haast hoping to skip around my itinerary before a front moved in, but found the weather was moving faster than predicted. It just wasn't safe to fly the fixed-wing through the Main Divide to Te Anau as planned, so Dave Saxton helped out by flying Marc and me to an idyllic little slice of paradise called Gunn's Camp in the Hollyford Valley. This meant it wasn't too far for the Te Anau pilots to drive through and meet us.

It was a really interesting flight in, taking us along the main alpine fault through the Duncan and Pyke river valleys and over Lake Alabaster. Dave loves this area best, and gave us a running commentary on all sorts of points of interest, such as the Red Hills, which are — get this — red, and mysteriously devoid of vegetation. Somewhere up there, Dave reckons, is the lost ruby mine reported by prospector William 'Arawata Bill' O'Leary in the nineteenth century. And Sax also claims to know where there is a pickaxe sunk in a tree that marks the vicinity in which another prospector cached a boot full of gold. It's not uncommon for him to head off up into this country to chase up his latest hunch on where those fabled treasure troves might happen to be.

We descended into the Hollyford Valley, the massive Humboldt and Darran mountains on either side, and then down onto Gunn's Camp, the site of a former relief labour camp established during the Great Depression. It's an awesome place, known for its tranquillity, and is a haven for greenies and them what needs a bit of peace and quiet.

For an hour on that particular day, it was more like *Apocalypse Now*. Dave loudly swooped into the camp and landed amongst the tents. Many went flying, exposing a bunch of semi-naked folk in various compromising positions. Wocka-wocka-wocka... And there was another one! Followed by the whine of four-wheel-drive transmissions in low gear, and a jeep or two dragging dust clouds into camp before braking heavily.

I set up in a small hut while a bunch of rather uncouth men surrounded it, yelling and laughing and using language that deviated from the Queen's English as they filled in their rather crumpled medical examination questionnaires with grubby, work-stained fingers. It was a hoot!

By the time some of the punters had retrieved their tents and set them up again, we were ready to go. I felt a twinge of pity for those who had their temporary shelter blown away all over again as we lifted off. All I could do from the passenger's seat was wave and shrug my shoulders in a gesture of sympathy.

This, I reflected, is what it was all about: spending time in the greatest place on earth with a bunch of good bastards.

One evening, as the autopilot took care of business and I was sitting, sipping a cuppa and twiddling my thumbs at 10,000 feet en route from Hokitika back to Palmy, I pulled out my abacus and crunched a few numbers. I was quite surprised to find that over

90 per cent of the pilots I examined were within one hour ten minutes' flying time of base at Palmerston North. The remaining 10 per cent or so were two to five hours' flying time away, with the most distant at Stewart Island. Yet I would charge a Stewart Island pilot on whom I did a medical the same as someone who yawned, scratched his nuts and walked across the road to the medical centre at Bulls. If I were the bean-counting kind, this might have bothered me: I certainly wasn't going to get rich out of doing my tours to the Deep South. But let's face it, I ain't counted a bean in me life, and the whole point of working in the Southern Alps was so Marc and I could live the lifestyle to which we had become accustomed.

By now, word had sort of spread about what I was doing with the Not-So-Royal Bulls Flying Doctor Service, and I was asked to speak to various groups, such as the Lions, Rotary and whomever. I spun a few hunting yarns and talked about my work a bit, and I also began dropping in a few bits of advice on how a man might live a healthy lifestyle.

Of course, for the most part, I was preaching to the converted at this sort of show. They were mostly populated by lean, mean, muesli-munching yogic types who had had their doctor poke a finger up their ring-piece at one point or another, so not much of it was news to them.

But part of my work as a rural GP was to sign death certificates, and it had not escaped my attention that a lot of the good bastards I was consigning to the great beyond were quite young, and they were dying of shit they didn't need to be dying of, especially at that age. There was an obvious contrast between the slobs who overpopulated the Bulls Medical Centre waiting room and the paragons of health and beauty I would examine for pilot medicals. The difference stems from pilots having more than the usual vested interest in looking after their health, as losing their right to fly usually meant losing their livelihood. The rest of the population, on the other hand, didn't seem to give a shit, especially the men. I used to idly wonder if there was some way of reaching this type of bloke, telling him to get off his fat ass, do a bit of exercise, cut the crap out of his diet and get himself checked out by his friendly GP from time to time.

One day, as I signed yet another death certificate for some unhealthy bastard gone too soon, it hit me like lightning. I needed to launch a public awareness campaign, where I would do presentations — long on hunting yarns and short on political correctness — to the kind of Kiwi who needed to hear the message.

It just so happened that in 2002 I caught up with Rob Neil, the editor of New Zealand aviation magazine *Pacific Wings*. He seemed pretty impressed by me and my operation, and apparently he was also moved by my passion for the subject of men's health, too, because he rang me one day soon afterwards and asked if I'd like to do a medical column for the magazine.

Why, yes, I told him, I would. And then I smoothly laid out my terms and conditions. I didn't expect a bean in return, and not because I didn't count them: instead, I would like to retain ownership of the material so that, in due course, I could compile it and publish it as a book that I would call (drum roll) ... *Fitness to Fly for Healthy Bastards*.

Rob was cool with all of that, so I began to set pen to paper. The Healthy Bastards campaign was born.

Soon enough I began to get invitations to speak to the kind of group I wanted to reach. Anywhere where there was a captive audience of the adipose, she'll-be-right minded — the average Kiwi bloke, in other words — was ideal. When I was asked by the manager of Manawatu Prison to come and do a preso there, I was only too happy to agree. It was literally a captive audience of men who (for the most part) lacked the advantages of education and the sorts of life choices available to the well-heeled.

On the big day, Marc and I went into the prison and set up all our audiovisual gear. Man, prisons are horrible places. Everyone who ever wrote an angry letter to the editor complaining that we're too soft on prisoners should go and experience the sights, sounds and smells within those mean concrete walls.

We had a bit of a stunt planned. With the permission of the prison manager, Marc flew me in and set the chopper down in the exercise yard of the maximum security section of the prison. To say we were given a rapturous welcome is an understatement!

In the hall, the audience was already assembled, listening to the prison band. Boy oh boy, could they play! Their rendition of Santana's 'Black Magic Woman' had the hairs standing up on the back of my neck.

With the crowd nicely warmed up, it was soon my turn. My preso went down pretty well, and I couldn't help noticing that Marc was the most popular he had ever been. It seemed everyone with a bit of a stretch ahead of them wanted to sit next to the chopper pilot and talk him into taking them for a little ride.

At the end of my talk, I took questions. Quite a few of them were pretty dorky, even if they got a few laughs. But when one heavily tattooed hand went up, everyone fell quiet. You could tell that this guy was the kingpin, and that you didn't fuck with him. He asked his question, and I answered it respectfully. He listened, nodded and everyone breathed again. Then they went right back to asking lame-arse questions.

It was a blast! At the end, as we made our way out to the chopper, we had plenty of offers from inmates keen to keep us company on the flight out. It was such a buzz, and it was a good feeling to have got the message across to those guys.

As if I needed a reminder of how important the message was, I asked Marc to drop me off at a client's place on the way back to base. This bloke was a very experienced pilot, with more than 40,000 commercial hours under his belt (not that there's much room under his belt, because he also happens to be a big fat bastard). I was always having him on about his weight, but he used to assure me that it was nothing to do with his diet or his lifestyle. It must have been some quirk of his genes or his physiology, he reckoned. All those old excuses.

Yeah, I used to say, right.

On this particular day, he wasn't expecting me. As I grabbed the folder with his medical results in it from behind the chopper seat and ran, stooped, out from under the rotors towards his house, he came out shoving the last of a cream doughnut into his gob, around which were the unmistakable signs of the recent greedy consumption of a pie.

'Got you, you bastard!' I roared, and he knew he was sprung.

As busy as we were, Marc and I made sure we kept our eyes firmly on the prize and went hunting as often as we could. He was turning out to be a terrific hunter: a good outdoorsman, fit and at home in the bush and the mountains, besides being a good shot and blessed with unbelievably sharp eyes.

We were becoming rivals, as well as mates. I still remember, without jealousy, the day Marc shot his first stag, or should I say, stags, because he actually shot two within 12 hours of one another. The first hunt was a bit dodgy. It happened on the edge of Dave Saxton's farm at Haast. Marc and I had just arrived in the jeep on our Deep South aviation medical round for the month, the weather being too bad to fly. The plan was that after I had done a few medicals at the Haast Aerospace Research Centre, we would overnight at Dave's place. Staying with the Saxtons was always the highlight of these trips — Lisa or Debbie were often about, and they really knew how to cook. I was through with the medicals about an hour before dusk and I happened to mention to Dave that it was time Marc got to shoot a stag.

'What d'you reckon's the best way to make that happen?' I asked.

Dave slapped the fronts of his thighs and clapped his hands together.

'Let's go!' he hollered, and a minute later we were stuffed in the three-seated Heliventures Hughes 300. I was in the middle seat while Marc was on the outside with the door off cradling my .270. I made sure he was very well strapped in! As we lifted off, Marc had a massive grin from ear to ear; he was so excited he could hardly speak. Within a few minutes we were skimming along the farm perimeter looking for one of the many fallow deer that had escaped Dave's rather holey deer fences.

'There's one!' yelled Marc, pointing forward and down.

The chopper banked sharply and put us over the unfortunate young stag. Marc lined it up with the .270.

Boom!

No luck. Boom. Again, then again and again. Six shots later, the stag was still hopping about like a mad jackrabbit in heat, quite the picture of health. It all got a bit messy as I tried to thumb fresh .270 cartridges into the magazine while Dave flung the chopper this way and that trying to keep it over the animal.

Marc slapped the magazine back in the rifle, worked the bolt and poked it back out into the air between us and the stag. It darted left and right, around and over bushes at great speed, but Dave managed to keep us in a good firing position, cussing and yelling the whole time as I hung on for dear life.

Boom! Still the animal bounced around.

'Fuck!' I yelled at Marc above the roar of the engine and the wind. 'Put the bloody cross hairs on it.'

'I am!' he yelled back. 'It just won't keep still.'

'D'you blame it?' I shouted, and he did that duck and smirk thing in reply.

Boom! Boom, boom, boom, boom!

Finally, five shots later, the animal fell to the ground.

'Phew,' I muttered, while Marc let go with a 'yahoo!' that most of Haast must have heard.

We landed near the very dead deer which turned out to be only a very young spiker. Marc wasn't worried: he was just rapt to have finally shot his first stag. While using a helicopter is sort of cheating — just ask any high-country farmer — it's not easy, especially when the rifle is about as big as you are. I was especially proud of the way he kept his cool throughout the whole wild exercise.

The very next morning, Marc and I got up at four o'clock for a quick breakfast of Dave's famous poached eggs with Worcestershire sauce, then we headed off in a big rush. We had pilot medical appointments at Fox Glacier and Hokitika planned for later in the day, after which we'd do a runner for Picton so we could catch the Interislander across the Strait to Wellington at six-thirty and then home to Palmy. With nine hours' driving and two hours' worth of medicals on the menu, we figured we had a spare hour up our sleeves to have a quick look up one of the side creeks of Lake Moeraki for a deer. After a big goodbye to our hosts, we screeched out of Dave's drive in a shower of flying gravel and made double-quick time to the creek. Half an hour later we arrived, grabbed the rifle and began picking our way up the steep, rocky creek bed. There was a well-grassed cliff face where we were hoping we might find a few deer.

The morning light was starting to sneak over the surrounding mountaintops as we huffed and puffed upwards. It's a funny time of day, because the dim light can turn trees and boulders into the image of deer. But on this particular morning we didn't have time to be dicked around by Mother Nature's little tricks of the light: we just kept moving fast to get to the big slip.

We timed it perfectly. As we came around the last bend in the creek, the light was bright enough to clearly make out the deer dotted up the slope.

'There's three,' whispered Marc without a moment's pause.

I squinted, counted and chuckled.

'You're bloody right.'

Due to a lucky combination of the wind blowing in our face and the noise of the stream muffling our boots crunching on gravel, the deer weren't aware of our presence. I handed the rifle to Marc and he knelt down, resting it on a large rock. He closed the bolt, lined up on one of them and . . . Boom! The deer nearest to us instantly crumpled and rolled down the slip like a sack of spuds.

'Wow, you got the bastard with one shot!' I yelled.

The other deer did a runner as we scrambled up to the base of the cliff to admire Marc's prize. It was a six-pointer stag in velvet with a very good skin. We skinned out the deer, grabbed some meat and hurried back down to the jeep. Exactly an hour later, we were on the road again heading for Fox Glacier, laughing and chattering. You couldn't have shut Marc up with a roll of gaffer tape. He was so excited because it was his first real stag — proper stalking, rather than death from above. As he was bollocking on excitedly, I remembered my first buck up on Arete and I felt a huge surge of pride that my son had got to experience the same thrill. He was only fucking twelve! Of course, as his trainer I took full credit, but I wondered if I was actually more proud of him than I had been of myself. I remember thinking: this is living!

=

Marc got me a beauty one day. We had popped into Jojo (another of Sir Tim's sons) and Annabel Wallis's place to the west of Lake Wanaka to stay the night. We had the idea that we would shoot up the hill to barrel ourselves a few chamois before we started our working day.

After a monstrous breakfast, Jojo dropped us off on a high ridge up behind their house on the Wallis family's Minaret Station. We gathered our gear together and started to climb to a high, snow-covered peak that looked down on the Albert Burn, with a view to settling down up there for a while to glass the faces below for a trophy chamois buck.

I had taken care to pack my prize set of Swarovski EL Range 10x42 binoculars. I had got these off a patient at Bulls called Mike, a really cool guy who was a hunting guide. Knowing my interest in hunting — it must have been all the antlers and hunting photos on the medical centre wall that gave me away — he had proudly shown me this set of binos during a consultation at the Bulls Medical Centre. It was my sad duty to diagnose a chronic illness that didn't have the best outlook. I didn't think he'd last more than a year, so I craftily suggested that if he gave me them binos, I would treat him for free for the rest of his natural life.

'Deal!' he said.

The binos were mine!

The only problem was that the bastard just wouldn't die. In fact, 10 years later, he's still alive — some deal that turned out to be — and when he turns up at the surgery in Bulls, we still laugh about it.

'Die, you bastard,' I say, after every consultation.

'Fuck you,' he chuckles, as he wanders out past reception without reaching for his wallet.

'Well, you can't win 'em all,' I mutter to myself.

But in the end, he's an amazing hunting guide and this world would be a poorer place without him.

Marc led me plodding up the ridge. Not only was he fitter, but he was also keen as mustard to bowl over a big fat chamois.

Then, for some reason — maybe he slowed down to tie up his boot laces — I got in front. I was creeping along a small, razorback ridge when I suddenly found myself looking down a steep slope onto a big chamois buck enjoying a leisurely breakfast of alpine plants.

Slowly, deliberately, I swung my daypack off, fitted the butt of my .270 to my shoulder and put the cross hairs of the scope on his chest. Boom! He was mine.

Marc came running up with disappointment etched all over his face. It wasn't often I got one over him and I knew he wanted to bag that first chamois real bad. I held the pose as he approached, rifle to my shoulder. I slowly lowered it, held his eye with mine and pulled back the bolt to eject the spent cartridge. As it tinkled off the rock, I drawled, Dirty Harry-style: 'Yeah, baby! I got 'im good. Ya have a problem?'

Marc had been looking really pissed off, but then his expression changed.

'Nah,' he said casually. 'Reckon you're the one with a problem.'

I narrowed my eyes, not understanding.

'Whaddyamean?' I rasped. 'Ya reckon I'll run outta ammo with all these chamois about, baby? Reckon I should use one bullet to shoot 'em in twos from now on, eh?'

Marc was grinning by now.

'Nup. Your problem,' he said, enjoying himself, 'is that you kicked your daypack off the edge of the cliff on the other side of the ridge, you dickhead. Y'all just go on down and look for it, now, and I'll just mosey on ahead, eh.'

He laughed, gave me a wink and headed off up the hill. I then spent the next two hours working my way down the cliff searching for my daypack. It wasn't hard to find. All I needed to do was follow the trail of gear that had fallen out of it as it tumbled down. And, of course, the one bit of gear I couldn't find was only my prize set of Swarovski binos!

To add insult to injury, Marc later shot a real beauty chamois buck, and didn't he let me know about it!

Bad day at the ranch for Davie today. Good day for Marc.

Once we got back to Bulls, Mike the Hunter also had a good day, because I was silly enough to tell him what happened. He gives me a chuckle every time I see him at the medical centre these days.

'How's your deer-spotting going, Dave?' he yells with great mirth.

'Die, you bastard,' I reply.

CHAPTER 12

TRIALS AND TRIBULATIONS

'Wow! One of those is a trophy for sure!' yelled Marc over the intercom as he glassed the Himalayan tahr on the sheer, dark 4000-foot cliff face running down from the top of Mount Sefton.

Watching tahr run wild and free over precipitous South Island rock faces, the wind flicking through long, thick winter coats, a sickening plunge to a horrible death just a misstep away . . . it's one of the most awesome sights in nature.

'How the hell does anything live up here?' I mumbled to myself.

A few seconds later, Marc lowered his binoculars, his eyes gleaming.

'Wow. I'd love to get that big one in my scope.'

'Yeah, me too,' I replied. 'But if you shot one, it'd be a hell of a job retrieving the carcass!' He nodded in agreement.

I risked a glance at the spot he'd seen the tahr, but the aircraft was moving so quickly all I saw was a tawny blur. We were getting dangerously close to the grim, grey cliff and the wind was throwing the plane about, so I decided my time was better spent focusing on the aircraft controls.

We were heading south at 8000 feet, high above the Karangarua River and just west of mighty 10,300-foot Mount Sefton. Against the enormity of the landscape in the Southern Alps, you feel a sense of your own insignificance, of the incomprehensible forces that created this mass of twisted rock, rushing water, snow and ice. For all of our grand schemes and dreams, we're of no more significance than the tiny little West Coast sandflies. You can't help but be reminded of your own mortality here and the fact that we're only visitors on this planet.

It can all be over in a single, unexpected instant.

Marc and I were sharing one of our best moments, where we were just sitting in silence and being together. I'm sure he was thinking exactly what I was thinking.

As I banked the aircraft over yet another razorback ridge, I heard Harvey Hutton making a radio call on 119.1 MHz, a frequency used for traffic flying in and out of unattended aerodromes. I couldn't make out what Harvey was saying, but I caught the words: 'I hope they're OK.'

Then another voice that I recognised came on. It was Debbie Saxton from Haast, and she sounded concerned.

'They are well overdue,' she said.

That got my attention, so I butted in and asked Harvey what was up.

'Sax and Geoff haven't come back. I'm just about to head off and see if I can find out what they've done to themselves,' he replied.

I reminded him that I had a comprehensive medical kit on board. That was stretching the truth, but I had something more than a few Band Aids. Both of us also knew that Harvey hated the sight of blood, so I suggested we meet somewhere so we could go looking for the boys together. He was into that, and so without further ado I put ZK-Really-Jolly-Good into a full-power dive, heading directly for the Haast airstrip 10 minutes away.

Harvey's Hughes 500D looked all revved up and ready to go as I dropped over the fence on short final (the last part of the approach to land) coming into Haast. Marc and I jumped out as soon as the engine had shut down. I grabbed my medical bag, gave Marc the thumbs up and hopped into the waiting chopper. Marc stayed behind to commandeer the phone and make courtesy calls to the pilots who had medical appointments with us that morning over in Wanaka.

As we swooped into the air and clattered towards Barn Bay, Harvey told me that, according to Debbie, Geoff, Dave and a couple of others had gone walkabout in Dave's chopper early that morning to maybe check out a bit of the local geology and shoot a few deer south of Barn Bay. They had been due back long before now, and she hadn't been able to raise them on the radio.

Once he'd briefed me, we were both quiet. Both of us had attended fatal aircraft and motor vehicle accidents, so we sort of knew what to expect if the worst had happened. But it would be harder than usual, because if we did find a helicopter wreck on this beautiful, calm West Coast morning, it was our mates who were involved. It's funny where your mind goes in situations like this. You find yourself thinking stupid stuff like: 'I hope it's him and not him, because he has a young family whereas he's an old bastard...'

Harvey kept us low to stay out of a slight southerly headwind that might have slowed us down. Before long we were skimming up and over the Cascade Plateau, a strange, broad-topped range of hills that runs from the high mountains of the Main Divide in the east to the sea in the west. The plateau has always fascinated me, because beneath its light covering of tussock, you can clearly see the contortions produced by the movement of the tectonic plates on either side of the main Alpine Fault.

My guts lurched as Harvey made a rapid dive into the wide and well-grassed Cascade River valley. We swung west and for a few minutes followed the winding and twisting Cascade River in its broad, swampy course until we arrived at the coast just south of the river mouth.

'Keep your eyes peeled,' Harvey said over the intercom. He was sure the fellas would have been working south of this point, so we began seriously scanning for a wreck. We ran south about 100 feet above the wave line; from here we could see the beach, get a good look up the deep gullies that plunged inland and also see about 500 metres out into the ocean. If Dave's machine — the same as the one we were flying — had come to grief along this wild stretch of coastline, we thought we'd have a pretty good chance of spotting it.

Barn Bay airstrip flicked by.

'Fuck,' we both muttered. There were no aircraft on the ground. We had half expected to see Dave's chopper sitting there with a bunch of people locked tight in a bullshit session. Both Dave and Geoff loved to gossip with the locals, so it wasn't hard to imagine they had been held up at a place like this. All it would take is someone to mention the Department of Conservation and you'd be lucky to get a word in edgeways in a week of trying. We pressed on south with heavy hearts. It was beginning to look like the worst had happened.

Sure enough, a few minutes later, Harvey spotted something in the small dry bed of Callery Creek about three nautical miles south of Barn Bay. We wheeled around to investigate.

'Shit,' we said in unison. There it was, the unmistakable wreckage of a green Hughes 500D lying on its side, full of dents and surrounded by a very twisted set of main rotor blades. There was no movement or signs of life, apart from a large blue tarpaulin spread out on the ground near the wreck beneath which a couple of long humps could be seen.

We exchanged glances. Harvey was pale and I could see the same question in his eyes that he doubtless saw in mine. Two bodies. Which of the boys had been killed?

Harvey set us down about 100 metres away from the wreck and we both jumped out to head reluctantly towards the tarp and the two motionless humps. Halfway there, Harvey suddenly stopped in his tracks.

'Right. You go and check it out,' he said, with the air of a Prussian general directing Private Dave Baldwin, Iron Cross and Oak Leaves, to investigate a minefield.

I grabbed a large stick and slowly walked up to the blue tarpie. I took a deep breath and flicked up one edge, expecting to see a couple of feet poking out.

Nothing.

I lifted a bit more and to my great relief, I saw a couple of large packs stowed underneath.

'Yahoo!' I yelled in relief, letting the tarpaulin fall back.

'What are you on about, you wanker?' Major-General Hutton yelled back, giving me an evil look.

His attitude soon changed after he'd run on over and seen for himself what was under the tarpaulin.

'Phew,' he said, with great relief. We gave each other a spontaneous high five to mark the sudden lifting of the tension, then we started to scan the vastness of Fiordland National Park.

'I wonder where the silly bastards have gone?' Harvey spoke for both of us. Then: 'I bet they've gone to Beanie's. Let's look for tracks.'

It didn't take us long to find a set of fresh boot tracks in the sand that fitted with four men heading south in the direction of the Gorge River mouth, and home of Robert ('Beansprout' or Beanie for short) Long and Catherine Stewart. So, with great relief, we hopped back into the chopper and followed the tracks to the Gorge River airstrip. There were the boys, all alive and well, supping on bush tea and eating scones freshly made by Catherine on her bush stove.

We got the story of the crash — greatly exaggerated by now, of course — with everyone talking fast and loud as Mr and Mrs Beansprout doubtless wondered what had happened to the peace and solitude they'd come to Fiordland to find. We hung around for another half an hour while our nerves settled down. Then we all packed into Harvey's chopper and headed back to Haast, where Debbie and the rest of the Saxton clan were waiting in great relief. Harvey dropped me at the Haast airstrip where

Marc was patiently waiting. He'd already preflighted the plane; we waved them all goodbye as they lifted off for home.

The pressure to get to Wanaka was off because Marc had rung all the pilots and rearranged all of our appointments. I spent the next 10 minutes filling Marc in on the close call Dave and the boys had had, fluffing it up a bit, as bushmen are obliged to do. In my version, the boys were suffering and dying. Time was of the essence — blood loss, shock— and it was touch and go . . .

'Bullshit,' Mark judged with a wry smile.

Both of us then hopped into ZK-Really-Jolly-Good and we took off up the Haast River valley bound for Wanaka via Haast Pass. This was one of our favourite scenic legs to fly, and we were soon absorbed in trying to spot a big stag that might have wandered out onto one of the many slips that can be found on either side of the valley. When we got to the junction of the Haast and Landsborough rivers, I banked left and we headed up the Landsborough River valley for a gander. We soared up past Harper Flat and over the steep Landsborough Gorge before diving down towards the Creswicke Flat Hut, nestled on the flats just up from the gorge and under the fearsome Brodrick Pass 4000 feet above us.

'Remember that time . . .?' we said to each other.

'And how about that time when . . .'

=

In 2007, after hawking the manuscript of *Fitness to Fly for Healthy Bastards* around a total of eleven publishing houses, I decided that I was going to have to publish the thing myself. With the help of Wyatt & Wilson Print in Christchurch, along with Megan Foster tidying up the book, that's what I did. I printed 700 copies and it sold pretty well. Based on my *Pacific Wings* column, it sought to raise your average unhealthy bastard's awareness of the miracle that his body is and the care and attention it deserves to receive. I did this by referring to the experiences of a certain daredevil mountain helicopter pilot by the name of Gav McAvedy (any resemblance to persons living or dead is purely coincidental). But even more gratifying than the sales I was getting was when, at the urging of local writer Keith Butler, I de-pilotised it to make it more accessible to a general readership and it was picked up by a major publisher, Random House.

I cared less about the cash, the women and the fast cars that go with a major publishing contract: I reckoned I was onto something with the whole 'Healthy Bastards' thing. It seemed like an issue that really needed to be brought to the attention of the general public. I realised how deeply I cared and began hatching other schemes: sponsoring the local rugby competition, instigating a bush pilot's flying competition at Omaka (both bearing the 'Healthy Bastards' name) and then, who knew . . . but probably Hollywood, or at least a movie.

To this end, I fitted a GoPro to the tailfin of ZK-Really-Jolly-Good, to capture footage of a healthy bastard living an inspirational lifestyle. And I decided that in order to show that I was prepared to go outside my comfort zone, just as I was asking unhealthy bastards to venture outside their own, I would do something ballsy. I would jump out of a plane while its motor was still going and it was still answering to controls. Yep, I would do another tandem skydive and this time I would film it. I talked to Sarge at Skydive Fox Glacier, and he was enthusiastic about taking me up again. My mouth immediately went dry. There was nothing for it now.

After a few years of sterling service, our amazing administrator Flying Jeanie resigned and we had a big think about what sort of replacement we wanted. It wasn't an easy job, as Marc and I were a bit loose and made decisions on the run. What's more, the place was in a constant state of flux as I had the 'Healthy Bastards' tiger by the tail and Marc continued to work hard developing his own company.

Fortunately for us, Rosemary turned up. I met her in similar circumstances to Karen at the Bulls Medical Centre, in that she popped in for a consultation and we got chatting. Rosemary's kids had just left the nest so she was looking for a job, although she wasn't overly sure how to go about it. She'd seen our administration job advertised on TradeMe, but didn't feel she was up to it. I've quite often seen this low confidence level in women looking to get back into the workforce: everyone knows they're awesome except themselves.

'Why not come and manage the Not-So-Royal Flying Doctor Service with Marc and me?' I said.

Rosemary looked a bit taken aback, but she agreed and she turned out to be as awesome as I suspected. The three of us became a really tight team.

It was hard yakka in those days. The 'Healthy Bastards' campaign added to the long days and nights I was putting in at the Bulls Medical Centre and with the NSRBFDS. Marc was managing the aviation medical services — doing the finances, organising medical appointment times and setting up flight plans, all the while developing the helicopter company he'd long dreamed of, and which we had called Helicopters Manawatu Ltd. There was, in short, no time to fart about.

One morning, I met Marc at home around four o'clock to discuss the day's flight down south. After walking through the plan, he shot out the back door to his jeep and I shot out the front door to mine. We had two driveways at our house in those days, and they merged at the front of the house to join the street. We were so preoccupied with the day's plans and how little time we had to fit everything in that we both jammed our pedals to the metal. I registered a flash from my left just as he registered a flash from his right and then there was a big, hollow 'BANG!'. We both got out of our respective jeeps, looked at the large dents and uttered a 'Fuck!' before shrugging and heading off into the dark in opposite directions to get our jobs done. Just another day in the life of the NSRBFDS. There was no time to worry about a couple of dents. After all, the jeeps still worked fine.

On 4 September 2010, I was all ready to set off on another Deep South tour. After a night of uneasy dreams about falling out of planes and the chute not opening, the alarm went off as usual at 0345 hours. Sandi and I got up and did our well-oiled team thing: I got my gear together while she fired me up some breakfast and filled the old lunch box. After a wave from Sandi, I was off to the hangar where Marc was preflighting ZK-Really-Jolly-Good. The ungodly hour notwithstanding, I loved turning up to the NSRBFDS hangar after Marc had arrived because he would really have the place humming. The music would be on, the coffee pot brewing, the hangar lights sparkling and he'd be whistling some tune as he lovingly scrubbed up the Cessna.

It was business as usual until about 0435 hours when I wandered into Rosemary's office and rang Airways, New Zealand's air traffic control service, in Christchurch to file my flight plan to Hoki and Fox Glacier. Back when I was working as the doctor at RNZAF Base Ohakea, the Airways Corporation had a flight control centre located there. This meant New Zealand had two main flight control centres, with the other being in Christchurch. Then some bunch of rocket scientist bureaucrats decided, in the interests of cost saving, that they'd merge the two centres into one big one at Christchurch, citing that city's comparative safety and the low threat of natural disasters. In my view, along with many of the front-line controllers, the decision to close the Ohakea flight control centre was ridiculous.

Anyway, the bloke I was talking to on the phone seemed like a really cool guy and we joked a bit as I worked through the details of my flight plan, such as cruising altitude, airspeed, expected time of arrival and so on. I was just about to utter the very last sentence of the plan, whereupon it would be job done and I could get on with my day, when the guy at the other end of the phone went all nervous and strange.

'Shit,' he said. 'The fucking roof is falling in.'

'Come on,' I said. 'Just hang in there. I've only got a sentence to go.'

There was a short pause, then he shrieked: 'Airspace is cancelled! I'm outta here!' and the phone went dead.

'That's weird,' I said to Marc, as he wandered into Rosemary's office. 'The bloke from Airways has just lost his mind!'

We were a bit puzzled until a few minutes later when a news item came across the radio announcing what came to be known as the Darfield earthquake, the first of the big ones to hit the Canterbury region in a six-month period. With a magnitude of 7.1 it scared the shit out of the locals (including our mate at Airways), but because of a number of factors, including the aforementioned ungodliness of the hour, not many people were injured. Months of significant aftershocks followed and, on 22 February 2011, another big quake struck the city in the middle of a working day and killed 185 people.

I couldn't take off and fly into controlled airspace with an IFR plan until Airways gave me the required approval. It took about two hours for the team to get back in action, and the new person I spoke to naturally sounded a bit tense and uptight. But we got the job done, and I soon had the OK to take off on my Deep South trip, albeit a couple of hours later. No panic, though: Marc just had to reschedule the medical appointments I had lined up. We found the pilots always seemed to understand that if appointments were being changed it was because of things that were out of our control, such as the weather. Now we could add earthquakes to our list of good excuses.

I landed at Hokitika Airport. After doing five medical

examinations as quickly as I could, I headed off for Fox Glacier at full steam. I was more excited than usual about this visit: when I saw the Sarge (Rod Miller) standing waiting for me as I taxied in to the terminal at Fox, my palms went all sweaty. He helped me unhook the GoPro from the tailfin so we could get it ready for our tandem skydive.

Conditions were perfect and the plan was to do the deed immediately — they had a plane ready to go — but now that I was behind schedule due to the earthquake, I had less free time. The two pilots I had lined up for medicals had just turned up, as had a group of eight young tourists who were all nervously looking forward to their own jump. It made sense to let them jump in two groups of four, and I would try to get my own jump in later on in the day after I'd done my medicals.

I joked with Chaminda Senadhira, who was going to fly the Fletcher FU-24 and was refuelling it. I plonked my official Bulls Flying Doctor Service cap on his head and he flashed me his wonderful grin in return.

'Hey, Doc!' Adam Bennett, one of the tandem jumpmasters called. 'Has any bastard here got you a coffee yet?'

It was well known, wherever I went, that I am a man of simple needs.

'Nah,' I said. 'They're the meanest pack of pricks I've ever met!'

Even though they were behind their own schedule, Adam jogged over to the coffee cart that his partner ran and got me a flat white.

Meanwhile, the tourists were playfully debating who'd be in the first group to do the jump. When they'd got it sorted, the first group of four and their tandem jumpmasters started getting ready for the flight. The others ambled around talking and laughing amongst themselves. It was the usual friendly, happy atmosphere with great camaraderie.

Chris McDonald, another of the tandem jumpmasters, wandered over with the guy he'd be jumping with.

'Can you believe it? This guy's a vet, too!' Chris was a veterinarian when he wasn't jumping out of planes. 'I wouldn't trust this guy with my cat. Would you? And how safe do you feel, Doc, standing on an airfield outnumbered by vets?'

The tourist laughed.

As they were loading the aircraft, Mike Suter, another of the tandem jumpmasters, paused at the doorway and yelled to me: 'What's my vision like, Doc?'

I held up my Snellen chart for him to view from about 12 metres.

'You wouldn't see fuck all, you dumb bastard,' Sarge roared. Everyone laughed and the door of the Fletcher closed with a thump. I gave them a wave and climbed the stairs behind Nathan Healy to get on with his medical in my little clinic room.

I didn't see the aircraft's take-off roll, because I was concentrating on taking Nathan's blood pressure. I heard the engine's steady throb deepen into its usual bass roar as Chaminda gave it the gas down the strip.

'Shit!' someone yelled. 'What's happening?'

Nathan and I looked at each other, then we both looked out the door to see the aircraft climbing at a very steep angle. It then did a tight left-hand turn into a steep dive, before pulling out of it and flying straight and at low level directly back towards the airstrip.

Nothing struck me as amiss, but people started yelling.

'Go! Gooooo!'

I was puzzled about all the excitement. Why were they urging on a plane that was simply coming back to land?

Just over the fence, the aircraft suddenly flipped on its back in a rapid, left-wing drop-stall and plummeted a short distance into the ground with a 'crump' sound. A few seconds later, there was a massive fireball as its full load of kerosene fuel ignited. Nathan and I clattered down the stairs and jumped into his jeep, racing off to the crash site at five million miles an hour. We were the first there. We ran around the burning wreck from which tongues of burning fuel were extending, looking for anyone who might have been flung clear.

Nothing.

For me, the worst was yet to come. Over the roar of the fire, I became aware of a sound I had never heard before. I looked up towards the runway and saw a wave of people — the friends, relatives and workmates of everyone who had been aboard the plane — running down to the crash site. The screaming and wailing was unearthly, horrible. I had never seen an outpouring of grief like this before. It was made worse in that only a few minutes before, this place had been one of the happiest places I had known. Now the carnival atmosphere had been replaced by the most immense grief and suffering imaginable.

A few long, surreal minutes passed. Groups of loved ones cried, hugged and sobbed. The sadness and confusion was palpable. The fierce fire quickly burned out, leaving a smoking, charred mass of tangled metal. The only recognisable part of the aeroplane was the tail, which was relatively unscathed. After 15 minutes or so, a few individuals started walking away. Their body language — heads hanging, slumped shoulders, stumbling feet — spoke of resignation and indescribable grief.

Over the next three hours, the authorities turned up in force. The local volunteer fire brigade put out what little remained of the fire and a big contingent of police started circulating amongst the locals, taking statements. John Kerr, one of the co-owners of the skydive centre, had got news of the crash while in Christchurch, and somehow managed to get his Cessna 185 in the air and over to Fox. He came hurtling in and taxied to a rest amongst the police cars littering the runway. He climbed out of the plane and literally ran over to the police and his fellow skydivers. Poor John was as white as a sheet.

There was nothing I could really do. Soon after John arrived, I was allowed to take off. I got into the air and set a course directly for home. I felt a great need to be home and amongst the people I loved. I checked myself carefully to make sure I hadn't been so affected by the day's events that I was unsafe to fly, but beneath the awful grief I felt, I was calm. Perhaps that has something to do with the practice you get as a doctor, dealing with suffering and death as part of the everyday. I'd been doing it for 25 years by now. I wasn't hardened to it, but I think I had learned to accept it; death, they say, in the midst of life.

Still, it was a tough flight. My take-off took me directly past the crash site, and I flew out into the same airspace where something weird had overtaken another highly experienced, very competent pilot in a well-maintained aircraft. Then I climbed to 10,000 feet, looking directly over where they should have been only a short three hours before. There was a layer of stratus cloud over Fox

Glacier with the tops at about 8000 feet. This meant I couldn't see Aoraki/Mount Cook and its co-councillors until I had gone through a hole; and then, suddenly, there they were, presenting themselves to me in all of their awful majesty.

The next 10 minutes were spiritual. All that beauty remained, indifferent to the horrors I had left behind on the ground; it's funny how one moment can be so disconnected from the next. Landscape on this scale is slow to pass by; as I climbed and the mountains revolved slowly to my right, I thought about the good buddies I had just lost and those poor young tourists, who thought they were about to experience a highlight of their short lives. That made me think about everyone for whom death has come suddenly, and when they least expected it.

I set the autopilot and sat numb. I just needed to be home.

CHAPTER 13

AU REVOIR, MARC

The year 2012 wasn't the best for our family. Granny Olive was on the decline health-wise and it was so sad to see. She was an awesome woman, a tower of strength when we were kids, a maker-do and free spirit, the kind of natural rebel and unconventional role model that inspires kids to believe they can be anything they want to be. She was one of the greatest appreciators of Godzone you could ever hope to find.

Granny Olive was always interested in the natural history of New Zealand and, later in life, she developed an interest in the human history, too, especially Maori. She published over 11 books, including several children's books illustrated by her friend and kindred spirit Sheila Natusch, who absolutely shared her love of nature and those awesome stories from our past. I reckon she loved her three-volume history of D'Urville Island and Te Aumiti/French Pass the most.

In the 1970s, while researching the history of D'Urville, Mum heard a story about Hinepoupou, a young Maori woman who, abandoned by her husband, entered the water at Cape Terawhiti (the southernmost point of the North Island) and swam first to The Brothers — a group of rocks to the north of the Marlborough Sounds — and then on to D'Urville (then known as Rangitoto) where her home pa was. The 100-kilometre swim was supposed to have taken her five days. Mum was fascinated by the detailed descriptions of how she had gauged the tides and was completely convinced that the story was true.

To prove it, Mum was instrumental in arranging a recreation. In 1990, six pretty flash distance swimmers took four days swimming in relays to retrace Hinepoupou's route. The tides they encountered were eerily similar to those described in the old stories. Mum was on the support boat throughout and waded triumphantly ashore with the swimmers, wearing her trademark dazzling grin.

Besides her fame as a bush cook, Granny Olive was a born environmentalist — the scourge of possums — and was able to combine her two passions in the form of a pretty decent possum stew. Once I started visiting the West Coast, I was able to bring her back some of Bushman Pete's famous possum pies, which she loved. She absolutely idolised Pete and Justine Salter's free-spirited behaviour and their practical view of possums as less a pest than an abundant food source.

Mum was fiercely independent and opinionated. She wasn't that open to advice from friends, family or the medical profession.

I can remember in the 1970s, when I was a teenager, she proved herself well ahead of the American legal rort by trying to sue her poor, long-suffering GP for three million dollars! She was a tireless lobbyist and letter writer and lots of top people got a good and sometimes rough hearing from her, including then-prime minister Bill Rowling, Lord Richard Attenborough and any number of mayors, councillors and ministers of conservation. Despite the fact she had a go at anyone that crossed her, I couldn't help but respect her. She was often right, but just went over the top a bit trying to sort things out. She passed away after a short illness in mid-2012 and such was the nature of her illness, it was a blessing.

We buried Granny Olive with lots of mementoes of her time in the bush and the mountains. We shrouded her body in the hides of Marc's first stag, our chamois skin from the Waiatoto River hunt and lots of possum skins. One of the best photographs I have of Granny Olive is of her sitting companionably with Marc in the Gorge River. I took it from behind them, so you can't see their faces, but they are shoulder to shoulder and the angle of their heads tells you they are absolutely absorbed in their conversation. She was a great loss to us all, but with the benefit of hindsight, especially to Marc.

=

Around the same time, I went to Greymouth to present my views on the Fox Glacier skydive tragedy to the Coroner's Court. In my opinion, there had been a swift and shabby investigation into the crash, and it had concluded that the Fletcher had been overloaded and its centre of gravity had shifted after take-off, causing Chaminda to lose control. This was despite a set of tests showing that the Fletcher could still be flown effectively under the same conditions.

I was upset with the findings. Nothing could bring the nine people back, but I felt John Kerr, Robyn (Rod Miller's wife), his family, and many of the others involved needed a bit of support. It was good to chuck in my five cents' worth.

Also around this time, Marc's business, Helicopters Manawatu, was entering a critical phase. He had worked his ring off getting it up and running. He had leased a Robinson R44 from our old mate Bruce Nicholson and, with this machine, he could start generating some serious local charter work. Matt Newton of Precision Helicopters helped Marc big time by allowing him to operate under his licence and by giving him the mentoring he needed as a fresh-faced chopper pilot. Meanwhile, Marc kept working on his skill set, getting his fixed-wing CPL and IFR ratings. He was humming and hawing about maybe going to fly for the airlines, but we both knew his heart was in the mountains. We kept our fingers crossed that we'd get a good break, but in the interim he practised what old Stan had preached: work hard if you want those doors to open.

In mid-2012, we heard that the R44 Marc was leasing was going to be sold. It was time to take stock. Business had been slow: there wasn't the scenic and tourist work in Palmerston North that keeps chopper pilots busy in other parts of the country and, man, do helicopters cost a lot to run! It's not so much fuel or operating costs as maintenance; it seems every time you turn one on you have to turn it off, pull it apart and put it all back together again.

The new owner of the R44 was happy for us to continue the lease, but we knew the only way to really make the business profitable was to get our hands on a turbine chopper. Most organisations who charter choppers — like the Department of Conservation, with whom we wanted to develop business relations — demanded the use of turbine choppers due to the perceived safety advantage (there are fewer moving parts in a turbine engine) and their bigger load capacity. But the costs of leasing a turbine chopper were prohibitive. We considered calling it a day and had all but decided that Marc should shoot off to Aussie for a while to do his Airline Transport Pilot Licence (ATPL) examinations when the opportunity arose to lease a Hughes 500C — a fast turbine machine — for six months. We jumped at it, because this gave Marc a golden opportunity to see if there was any mileage in the chopper business. If it didn't work with this machine, then it just wasn't going to work. We decided that if the business hadn't proved profitable by the time the term was up, we'd let the lease go and dissolve Helicopters Manawatu. It was no biggie. Even if it happened, it wasn't going to cost us a lot of dough and Marc would have over 100 very good turbine helicopter hours under his belt. They would count towards the Australian ATPL examinations he had booked for February 2013.

Getting this turbine chopper on board took us to a different level and, over the next couple of months, Marc trialled a number of projects locally like heli-biking and heli-tramping. Otherwise he did a few local scenics and the boys at Helicopters Hawke's Bay put a lot of frost work — stirring the air above vineyards and orchards with the helicopter's rotors to prevent a frost settling — his way, too.

Six weeks after we buried Granny Olive, Marc and I started planning a four-day tour of the Deep South doing pilot medicals. It looked like it was going to be a bit of a mission because the long-range weather prediction wasn't good. It was always a matter of wait and see — the West Coast and Southern Alps are home to some pretty dynamic weather. But as the weekend approached, it became clear that the only fine day during the four-day period was going to be Sunday, 7 October. Calling upon our full expertise in the dark arts of the management of time and space, we devised a fiendishly complex, two-part plan that would enable us to get around everyone despite the shitty weather.

On the Saturday, Marc and I spent all day together ringing the pilots, sorting out their notes and preparing the equipment required to do the medical examinations. The next morning, I took off from Palmy at four o'clock and flew direct to Milford Sound where there was a queue of pilots lined up for their medicals. I was done by midday and as I flew north to Neils Beach, I could see the dirty weather biding its time out to sea. After ministering to the needs of the Neils Beach aviation fraternity, I skipped up the Coast to Fox to do it all again, then on to Hokitika.

The sun had sunk behind a pall of cloud to the west as I levelled ZK-Really-Jolly-Good off at 10,000 feet for the cruise home. It was pitch-black by the time I was over Cook Strait in the capable hands of the autopilot, and I was basking in a glow of accomplishment. The second part was going to be easier.

My phone tinkled to announce a text arriving.

'Cruising on the Interislander,' Marc wrote. 'Free!'

'Awesome,' I texted back. 'Drinking coffee at 10,000.'

'Bring on the South Island!' he replied.

'Yeah. See you in Christchurch,' I wrote.

I looked down at the inky blackness of the Strait to see if I could see the lights of the ferry, but I couldn't. All the same, the warm glow intensified. You couldn't ask for a brighter prospect than spending a couple of days in the company of a bloke like Marc. The fact he was my son just made it more awesome and all the better that he seemed so happy.

After a few hours' sleep, early on Monday morning I boarded a commercial flight bound for Christchurch from Palmy. I felt quite smug looking across to the western side of the Main Divide and seeing it all clagged in with cloud.

Marc met me at Christchurch Airport with the jeep and we set off west towards Mount Hutt. We talked good-natured bullshit, told off-colour jokes on the way and, of course, made the obligatory comfort stop on the Rakaia Bridge (though Marc was a bit more careful to look out for kayakers this time). From Mount Hutt, we scribed a big circle over the next two days through Omarama and Wanaka before returning to Christchurch on Tuesday night. We were both pretty tired by the time he dropped me off at the airport on Tuesday night, but we grinned at one another as we parted, both of us pretty pleased with ourselves. We'd had some good laughs with some great people and Marc was pleased he was off to spend the night with our good mate Chris Brown at

Picton before catching the ferry the next day.

I put in a couple of full days at the Bulls Medical Centre on the Wednesday and the Thursday. Meanwhile, Marc got back to Palmy on Wednesday evening and set about catching up with mates and his helicopter work. On Thursday night, after the medical centre had closed, I was back at the hangar at Palmy doing a couple of medicals when Marc showed up.

'Got a deer,' he told me.

A bunch of Waipukurau pilots were due to stage a dawn raid on us that Sunday, and we had talked about cooking them up some wild venison as a big treat.

'When did you find time to shoot that?' I asked.

'Nah,' he grinned. 'Maurice sorted it for me.'

Maurice was one of his best mates.

'Awesome,' I told him, as he headed off to drop the carcass with yet another good mate, Lance Hurley the butcher, who was going to prepare it for the barbie.

=

Next Friday, in the early hours of the morning, I was working in my little office at home when the jeep pulled in. Marc came in bearing a couple of coffees: my favourite — a Wild Bean Café trim cappuccino topped with cinnamon and with one sweetener, from the BP service station in Rangitikei Street. We talked about our plans for the next few days and shot the breeze a bit. I can't really remember in any great detail what we talked about. Marc definitely prattled on about his mate Ollie coming back from

South Korea, about flying his chopper and where his girlfriend, Rachel — who was heading for a trip to Vietnam — would be at the moment. He had a booze-up arranged for that night then big plans to do some hunting that weekend. After an hour or so, he swapped the gear in our vehicles over and then came back in to tell me he was heading off.

All of this is captured on the CCTV camera I have installed overlooking my desk and the window, through which we once caught in glorious Technicolor a burglar clambering in, fully vindicating the decision to install the camera. Running the video, I can see us talking, me and my beautiful son. I am sitting, facing the camera. He is standing with his back to it. Of course, I can't hear what we're saying and nor can I remember, but he must tell a joke, because in the footage, I laugh and he does that sideways duck of the head that he and Andrew always did.

I remember getting up as he went to leave and watching him disappearing into the gloom of the hall outside my office. Something made me call him back. I had forgotten to show him the newly framed certificate proclaiming me a Fellow of the Australasian College of Aerospace Medicine. I took it down for him and he held it for a moment or two, nodding.

'Looks bloody good,' he said.

'Yup,' I agreed. 'This is my future, buddy. Yours is that ATPL course in Aussie next year, eh.'

He nodded again — a happy nod — and handed the certificate back to me. I have relived this bit in my mind countless times. Then he walked backwards down the hall and, as he waved goodbye, he seemed to fade from sight slowly in the gloom of the hall, and then he was gone from my life forever.

THE FLYING DOCTOR

It was a busy day at the Bulls Medical Centre, as usual. In the middle of the afternoon, around half past three, a cop appeared.

'Doctor Baldwin, I need to talk to you,' he said. 'Someone has died.'

That's what policemen normally say when they come in. I was a bit stressed and I remember thinking: 'Fuck, not now. Surely this can wait?'

But something in his eyes told me this wasn't the usual call-out to go and certify the death of some poor old codger in a rest home.

I ushered him into a private room. He waited until I was sitting down and then he said: 'Marc is dead.'

There was a stupid pause — seconds, minutes, hours, who knows. Time doesn't mean much, sometimes.

Then he said: 'He shot himself.'

I remember thinking: What? I mean, what? This was never a scenario I had planned for in my life.

There was a knock and Dr Ken came in. He had exercised his uncanny talent for smelling a rat and wanted to know what the hell was going on.

'What's up?' he asked.

I heard my voice telling him what the cop had told me.

He turned pale.

'Fuck,' he said. 'You'd better get going and sort it all out.'

The policeman offered me a ride to Palmerston North. I had done this journey so many times in so many different states of mind and degrees of fatigue, but never like this. It was completely surreal. They say it's better to travel hopefully than to arrive, but this isn't true when the hope is false. I kept hoping it was all some ridiculous mix-up, some terrible mistake. But I knew; I felt that it wasn't. It was the hope that was ridiculous.

Everything — thoughts, emotions, questions — passed me by, clear and remote from me as though they were rolling by outside the windows of the police car.

'Where do you want to go?' the cop asked gently, as we arrived on the outskirts of Palmy.

'The airport,' I said. 'The hangar.'

This, the cop had told me, was where Marc had done it. The aviation medical centre was his hooch, his happy place, and at some point in the late morning he had sat down, loaded his beloved .270, put the barrel under his chin and shot himself. He had arrived at the centre and gone in and out, calling a cheerful hello to Rosemary on the way. He seems to have sat in his car outside for a while: there was cigarette ash on the dashboard, even though Marc never smoked. He came back inside and there is security camera footage of him walking up the stairs. You can see from his body language that he means business. People sometimes tell you that suicide is a cowardly act, but there is nothing but courage and steely determination in his body language. The report of the gun was heard all over the airport. Rosemary knew what it was and she saw bloody material on the floor of the hangar. She phoned her husband, who went upstairs and found Marc. Then they called the police, who promptly went to the airport at New Plymouth by mistake. Soon enough, the cock-up was sorted out and they arrived in force.

There were six or seven cops there when I arrived. I knew most of them. We nodded at one another and then I went upstairs to the mezzanine floor where Marc had ended his life. His body had been removed, but I spent about 10 minutes walking around up there before sitting and taking everything in. There was still a large pool of blood and scattered pieces of body tissue and a neat hole in the ceiling. Weirdly, I couldn't cry. I could only look and grapple with the enormity of it.

'You'd better take me to the morgue, eh,' I said to one of the policemen after I descended the stairs.

'Sure,' he said. 'Let's go.' I shook the hands of all of the policemen before we left. There was tension amongst the group, as all of them knew the bond Marc and I had shared which made this business all the stranger.

I know the morgue well. Over the years, I had signed many a dead person's death certificate and had even spent time here with Andrew after he'd been killed in the chopper accident many years before. I knew the cop who was on duty. He's a good bastard. He greeted me and I felt comforted that my boy was in his capable hands. I was shown into the concrete space with its cold, sterile lighting and there he was, my beautiful boy. He was in a body bag but the zip was undone. I felt a rush of emotion: I was happy, just so happy to see him.

Maori have a few clues when it comes to dealing with death. An important part of the tangi is what they call poroporoaki, where you have a yarn to the dead person, tell them what you're feeling. I didn't do it out loud, but that's what I did.

I had two overriding feelings during my precious final hour with Marc. It might seem strange but that time I spent with him was some of the best. I was just overcome with how hard he had worked to try to succeed. I felt that, like most high-achieving young men, he must have experienced one of those dark moments that can come on quickly. I'd had a few along the way, and I could remember the feeling well. I also remember that when it happened to me, somewhere deep inside my consciousness I knew that if I kept thinking this dark bullshit, it could take me. I rebelled, but I could understand how Marc didn't.

'Marc,' I thought. 'It could have happened to me, bro, so don't fret!'

The second feeling I had was a strong will to keep what we'd built together going and not to bail. I would be strong, not only to keep my family and friends together, but also to help us all celebrate who Marc had been and what he had done. One of the first things I did after the funeral was order a huge sign that changed the name of the Palmerston North Aerospace Research Centre to the 'Marc Baldwin Aerospace Research Centre'. That way, anyone who ever has anything to do with me or my family can see for themselves that we celebrate Marc David Baldwin every day of our lives. Likewise we are hoping, through our faith and our sincere efforts to get some sort of understanding about life, that we live in his presence until our journey in this reality ends.

We buried Marc at Foxton Cemetery. It turned out he had discussed death with a close friend, but it had been in the context of what would happen in the not unthinkable event that he crashed his helicopter. He reckoned he wanted to be cremated and his ashes scattered over the Maori Lakes where he, Granny Olive and I had shared so many wonderful times.

Although we didn't grant him this wish, Sandi and I got Geoff Robson to organise a flight up into the area of the Maori Lakes to get him a headstone. We lifted it out, and it was carved with Marc's name and dates and set over his grave. I go there every week and scrub it up. It's not a morbid thing: on the contrary, it's like an anchor for me. I use the time while I'm there to plan my week, just like we did every week at Café Brie in Palmy before he died. It's there I wrote my song to Marc, 'Message to my Son'. My good mates Kev Downing and Mahia Blackmore and their band put music to my words. It's now on YouTube for all to see and hear.

The lovely thing about that stone is that when I tip water on it to clean it, it comes alive and looks just the way it did when I saw it in the stream bed. When I sit there, I can look to the east to Arete and I remember the feeling I had when I shot my first stag. And that sets all those great memories spooling, so many of them featuring Marc.

CHAPTER 14

BEYOND THE MATERIAL WORLD

According to the radio, I'm good to go.

I open the throttle and adjust ZK-Really-Jolly-Good's position for take-off. A short roll and then I ease back on the yoke and there's that awesome swooping feeling of lifting into the air. I've flown nearly 5000 hours now; I've been flying for the better part of three decades, and I've never got over it.

It's a beautiful, clear Manawatu morning, or it will be when the sun gets around to rising. There are patches of mist lying over the dark ground. To my left, the Tararuas are etched against the lightening sky. I can see Arete towering in the sky, where I nailed my first stag.

'Nice to see you, mate,' I think.

Soon I'm over Foxton, where Marc is.

'Hi, buddy,' I say and dip a wing for him. There's not a day goes by when I don't give thanks for his part in my journey. Whether people realise it or not, that's what it's all about: the journey. We get to share it with others; some you choose, some you don't. If you're as lucky as me, you get to share it with some really good bastards. There's no telling how long their journey will intersect with yours, so the thing is to enjoy the ride while it lasts.

Some years ago, I decided that my life's work was to help others see their way clear to becoming healthy bastards. I wrote my books, I made my movie and I still continue to do my talks around the country and on the internet. People expect me to talk about physical health, about how you treat your body and how you look after it. These days, it probably doesn't surprise people that I also talk about mental health, because gone are the days when doctors recoil as their patients try and talk about their personal, emotional and mental life. But some people do seem surprised that I also mention spiritual stuff from time to time.

Ageing is like gaining altitude: as you climb, you get to see the lay of the land. As I've become older, I've also become more and more convinced that the thing the healthy bastards among us all share is that we believe there is something more than the here and now.

The first itty-bitty sliver of sun comes blazing over the horizon as I am abreast of Port Underwood and soon the day will start for everyone down there as well. By the time most people are starting their workaday round with a shit, shave and shower, I'm already on my final approach to Omaka.

When I taxi in, I see ZK-PRM, the Cessna 185 that belongs to my mate Cliff Marchant, is already there. Cliff is another legend of New Zealand aviation; he's done 25,000 hours, flying all sorts over 40 years, including Boeing 747s for Air New Zealand. He also runs a small airline with his sons, Pelorus Air, flying out of Omaka, and servicing the people of the Marlborough Sounds. Like most born pilots, he's never tired of flying.

As I shut down ZK-Really-Jolly-Good, Cliff ambles out onto the strip to meet me. As we're talking, the buzz of an approaching aircraft announces the arrival of ZK-CIQ, the tiny low-wing Piper Pawnee belonging to Pete Anderson. Pete has been flying for 40 years, too, and has clocked up some serious hours in his capacity as Marlborough's Flying Vet. He visits backcountry stations and offers advice on animal health and productivity.

With the Flying Vet and the Flying Doctor here, all we need is the Flying Accountant, the Flying Lawyer and the Flying Consulting Engineer to drop in and we've got all the professions covered.

The plan from here is to take off and spend the day exploring the backblocks of Marlborough. Business had already taken each of us all over the region, many times, but our plan for today is to pursue pleasure.

We all get in the air, cruise in formation down Cloudy Bay a way, then swing south by west to pick up the Awatere River, just a little trickle right now in its braided shingle bed amongst the dry hills that look like brown paper from the air, like a pie bag that's been screwed up in God's pocket. We buzz Black Birch Station, Frank Prouting's place, where Marc and I cut our teeth as a team shooting goats back in the day, and press on to Alan Pitts' Mount Gladstone airstrip, where we set down for a bit of a yarn. There's a haze of cloud hanging about, but you can already feel the ground getting ready for another beating from the sun. There's the smell of dew, cow shit and tussock, mingled with the tang of Avgas.

Bliss.

You'd think, given how much care and attention I pay to safety and how much dosh I've splashed out on bells and whistles to keep me aloft and alive, that I'd be afraid of death, but I ain't. Life is a journey and it has to end at some point.

As a family doctor with about 5000 patients in my practice, I am, more than most people, able to witness the human journey in action from beginning to end.

In the early days of my work in Bulls I would deliver babies and witness the joy of a new child arriving in this world. Many were what I describe as 'beautiful births'. (Mind you, many of these poor little kids' first view of life as they shot out between their mum's legs was my ugly mug, so I hope I didn't scar any for life!) Then I would not only be involved with these children and their families as they worked through their own personal journeys, but would also be there at the end for many of them.

As a doctor, I've sat next to many people as they ended their journey and many have had what I would call 'beautiful deaths', as they passed on to the next dimension in an almost serene fashion. Some of them were healthy bastards, some of them definitely weren't, and some of them were somewhere in between. Some of the best times I have spent with family members has been just after they died. All of us will face those moments one day.

Ever since Marc died, I have been more focused than ever on loving every moment of life. I don't fret too much about what comes afterwards, if anything really does. We've got no control over it. The key issue for me is that when I am on my own death bed and drifting off, I want to be able to look back on my life with pride; that I gave it the best go I could and that I didn't piss off too many people in the process. I want to die a good bastard. Marc wanted to die a good bastard, too, and this is what he wrote on the noticeboard near him just before he pulled the trigger:

DIED A GOOD BASTARD

This is now tattooed on my right shoulder, along with 'Eternal love to Malach Marc'.

I knew Marc better than anyone else because of the way we had intertwined our lives, and I believe that no matter what was going on in his mind just before he died, he truly was a good bastard. Something tipped him over, maybe one day we'll find out, but it's not important now that he's gone.

There have been some tough times since Marc passed away. It was hard for our family, but if anything, it tightened the bonds between Sandi, Niki, Anna and me. We all shared a determination to celebrate Marc and the time we spent with him, and that's what we've done. I've met other people who have survived the suicide of a loved one, but some haven't really survived at all. They've been torn apart by it. I was adamant that wasn't going to happen to me or my family. And I'm proud to say that it hasn't.

=

We land at Molesworth Station after checking out a couple of mountain strips on the way and have a brew. After 30 minutes of having a good old rant and bullshit session we take off over Ward Pass for Redgate, which is now part of Molesworth Station. We catch up with Jim and Trish Ward who run Molesworth and are gurus on the history of this historic bit of farmland. Boy oh boy, it's dry up here, with the dirt showing through the brown grass. Jim and Trish just shrug when I mention it. Molesworth has suffered droughts before and will again. In between, there will be rain, and sometimes, too bloody much of it.

From the Redgate strip we head up the Severn River into some of Jim Ward's favourite country. It's awesome, all right, with those great, frowning shingle fans walling in the browned foothills and golden tussock plains along the river itself. Chamois and deer are running all over the place.

We land on a strip in the alpine meadow at Tarndale, where there is an awesome historic building. It was built back in the day when a string of such houses was set up along the route stockmen used when droving sheep from Nelson through to North

Canterbury. There's a sad story about this place, though. In the late 1800s, a station hand named German Charlie revealed to his drinking buddies the private contents of a love letter he'd been entrusted with delivering to a woman who lived in Wairau Valley, purely to spite the man who'd written it. Deeply ashamed, the man murdered German Charlie and then killed himself. His last name was Augarde and his first name was — get this — Ivanhoe.

Cliff, Pete and I have lunch — billy tea and soup — and tell lots of lies. We laugh and tell each other how awesome it is to be out here, with the people we're with. And we're not lying about that, or even exaggerating. Good times, with good bastards. It was here that Cliff and his wife Diane got started eeling in the large tarns that dot the landscape. They'd catch tons of eels and Cliff would fly them to the eel buyer in Levin. Once the eels got out mid-flight and he had to do an emergency landing.

From Tarndale, we head down the other side of the Inland Kaikouras, checking out a good old Kiwi mountain airstrip at Bluff Station, tucked under Mount Major, before flying on past Quail Flat on Muzzle Station and landing at The Branch. We take a few piccies here: this place, with Tapuae-o-Uenuku towering above it, was Granny Olive's favourite mountain strip. Then we head back over to Frank Prouting's for a cuppa. During the descent into the Awatere Valley, Pete does a magnificent barrel roll as the sun is setting, out of sheer joy.

Fucken awesome.

Me and my family went on a couple of trips. They weren't meant to be quests or pilgrimages or anything like that, although we did visit the kinds of places people go to stare at their navels and ask themselves the big questions.

We did a bit of the Camino de Santiago in Spain, a traditional route (actually, there's a whole bunch of routes, all known by the same name) to the Santiago de Compostela Cathedral in Galicia, where St James is supposed to be buried. And when we were in Europe, I built in a little side trip to Poland so that I could go and take a look at Auschwitz.

I found both experiences wonderful and moving, and there were moments where I think I had glimpses of the spiritual realm, and, I hesitate to say, I know I experienced Marc's presence near the end of the Camino.

But I don't need to go so far to feel this way. I feel it when I'm at 10,000 feet up in the Alps, or picking my way up a scree slope towards the snowline, or walking softly through the damp quiet of the bush, or talking to someone who has had an insight into themselves, or just spending time in my real spiritual home, the Marc Baldwin Aerospace Research Centre.

These days, when you start talking about the spiritual side of life, people start checking their exits and edging away, as though you're a card-carrying, wacko-jacko fruitcake. But I know nutters, and I'm not one. I just happen to know there is so much more to life than just the material side of it. People come to this realisation in lots of different ways. Some find it in organised religion, but I don't. Some feel claustrophobic in churches and have an allergic reaction to being told what to believe, or to being fed what they regard as a bunch of bullshit stories, or all of the above, but they find it out there in the 'big blue'. I reckon that's easier to understand.

Maori have their own spirituality and I am aware of its power. When we built the Marc Baldwin Aerospace Research Centre, I had it blessed in both the common and garden Christian rituals, and also by a kaumatua, a Maori elder. And likewise, when I began gathering mementoes of good bastards who had gone, to build a shrine to fallen pilots, I asked one of my best buddies and kaumatua of Ngati Parewahawaha, Ray Blackmore, to do a bit of a karakia over it. Ray passed on four days later and, as far as I'm concerned, this only enhanced the spirituality of the shrine. There are little plaques to all of the ones I have lost on the shrine, and I have the medical notes of all the pilots who have passed stored right there, on site.

Further spiritual power was added to the place in 2015 when Bevan Climo made a mere pounamu for my good Maori mate Dr Pete Morrison. It is very special in that it is totoweka pounamu, 'blood of the weka', due to the red colour running through the deep-green stone. One day soon after this beautiful object was delivered, Dr Pete arrived to pick it up. His eyes alighted on the mere, he picked it up and for nearly two hours he just walked around the hangar, eyes blazing while reciting karakia. It was awesome!

Plus, of course, the most awesome, awesome dude I have known, Marc David Baldwin, shot himself upstairs a few years back and his blood soaked the wood of the floor. That made it a sacred place for me, just as it was Marc's hooch and hangout while he was alive. The hangar has become a place where I can feel close to him.

I don't know what my spiritual beliefs are — call me stardust, if you like — but I know they're there. I'll happily argue about it with every Muslim-cum-Buddhist-cum-Jew-cum-Bible-banging, fair dinkum Christian who has ears to listen and the gob and gumption to put it into words. But I treasure the glimpses I have had into the spiritual side of other people; I am privileged that they have shared them with me.

Because of them, it doesn't worry me that sooner or later it will be a case of finally setting course for the sunset. I know there's a bunch of good bastards waiting for me.

'Make mine a chardonnay,' I text Sandi. It's late evening, pretty much dark and I'm at 9000 feet and about to start a full IFR descent to Palmy. Conditions are perfect. What a day it's been.

I said my big goodbyes to Cliff and Pete and Frank in the mountain valleys of Marlborough, and now I'm almost home. Sandi will have a nice dewy glass of wine ready for me after I've set down on the tarmac, which will still be warm from the glorious sunshine all day.

We'll sit together, my soulmate and me, and drink our plonk in the dentist's chairs at the door to the hangar and watch the last light leave the sky. Tomorrow will probably be nuts, with lots of flying doctor and medical centre and 'Healthy Bastards' stuff to deal with. Bring it on.

We'll meet whatever challenges the new day brings with our usual blend of energy, humour, bad language and good intentions.

We'll be loose as, and we'll fuck stuff up (hopefully not too badly), but we'll get most of it right. And along the way, if we are true to ourselves, we'll love every minute of it, because here at the Not-So-Royal Bulls Flying Doctor Service, that's how we roll.

EPILOGUE

With my story told, I want to highlight two important lessons that I feel have given me strength and kept me in a positive frame of mind through thick and thin. The first is the importance of having quality time with those with whom you share your journey. Ernest Hemingway said: 'It is good to have an end to journey toward; but it is the journey that matters, in the end.' I love that. It couldn't be truer. The journey Marc and I shared, even though it was short, was of the highest quality, so for that I am forever grateful. Since Marc died, I have become even more focused on seizing the moment with the people I love and having quality time with them, creating memories that I can treasure, should they depart before me.

The second lesson I have learned is that the definition of a healthy bastard can't be measured only in a physical sense. There's much, much more to it. To be a healthy bastard it's important to recognise that there is something beyond the material world;

to develop a personal, spiritual journey in addition to keeping physically well, is the key to being a truly 'healthy bastard'.

A healthy mind goes hand in hand with a healthy body. However you attain this is totally up to you, but instead of sheltering from the deeply emotional experiences over the course of your life, try to recognise and embrace them, just as you would the physical trauma or afflictions you might suffer. Ignoring them and their symptoms will only cause more pain and hurt. Just as you would visit a doctor for a physical problem, visit your own spiritual place for mental health.

In my case it's the Marc Baldwin Aerospace Research Centre, but it could be anywhere with personal meaning. Embracing the concept that there is something beyond the material world, however it appears to you, will enrich everything you do.

With that, hopefully you've enjoyed and been entertained by the stories in this book, but I also hope I've given you a few ideas and helped you out on your journey through life, because, believe me, it's something to be treasured and celebrated.

ACKNOWLEDGEMENTS

I will make this short and sweet because if I thank everyone who has truly helped me in making this book, I would be here all bloody day!

Those who I would like to thank can be grouped into five categories:

Firstly, the obvious place to start is with my family. Particularly Granny Olive, who not only brought me up in an environment where writing things down was a way of life, but also gave me the genes to have the balls to develop an opinion and stick with it. Sandi — wife, mother and soulmate — has supported Marc and me through everything, and her proofreading has given some respectability and sense to these pages. Then there are Niki and Anna, who are pillars of support and henchmen to be relied on through thick and thin.

Secondly, my buddies in Bulls who helped me form the Bulls Medical Centre, which is the platform from which Marc and I could make the dream of the Bulls Flying Doctor Service come true. Graeme Platt, Julie Ellery, Karen Greer and Dr Ken Young are just so cool!

Thirdly, my Bulls Flying Doctor Service buddies who helped make it happen. Neil Mathieson, the master avtech; Dougal Watson, CAA's Principal MO; and, of course, Rosemary Edmonds. Bush pilots and true free spirits Dave Saxton, Dick Deaker, Toby Wallis, James Scott, Murray Bowes, John Kerr, Rod Miller, Russell Gutschlag, Geoff Robson, Malcolm Walls, Penny MacKay, Frank Prouting, Chris Brown, Ray Patchett, Ritchie de Montalk, Gordie MacPhee, Maurie Rowe, Mike Bryant and Ian Wakeling. And, on the spiritual line, thanks to our good mates Ray Blackmore, Bevan Climo and Pete Morrison.

Fourthly, to the Penguin Random House folk. It's important for fledgling authors to recognise that if they get involved with the big boys of publishing they are part of a big machine. When I finished the first manuscript of this book, measuring 75,616 words, in January 2016, I thought it was a masterpiece — silly boy! Alex Hedley, as the non-fiction publisher, guided editor John McCrystal on the job to reorganise the whole thing, add a bit and then get me to write a whole lot more to fill in the holes. The manuscript was then given to a higher-level editor, Anna Bowbyes, to further tidy it all up, along with further demands on me to add this or that. In the end, exhausted, I recognised that their professionalism has really added to the story and made it much more readable, without the manuscript losing the important messages I wanted to get across. Rebecca Simpson then added her promotional magic to get the book out there to the shops. Thanks so much, and it's a real honour to be part of

ACKNOWLEDGEMENTS

such a well-oiled operation.

Lastly, thanks to the Big Guy in the Sky for organising my birth in such an awesome country as New Zealand, with its mountains, heaps of deer, freedom and great opportunities. Likewise, thanks boss, for giving all of us that special 24 years we spent with my son and 'bro' Marc. The only way I feel that I can personally repay the Big Guy in the Sky for this privilege is by trying to be a good boy and a follower of 'the way' — not easy when one is naturally 'bad to the bone'.

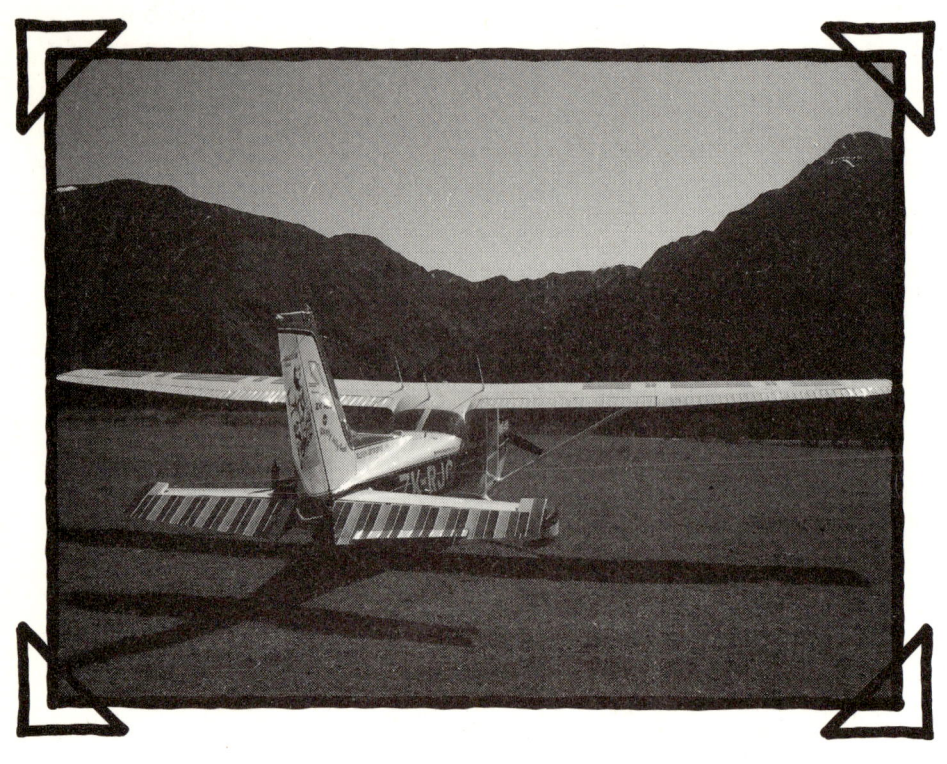